You Can Beat the Odds is a tested, inspirational "must" for any health collection. —*Midwest Book Review*

This book is *alive*! Brenda Stockdale combines reviews of cutting edge science with her rich experiences working with patients who manage to thrive in the face of overwhelming illnesses. It is fun to read and contains practices that *anyone* can use to benefit their health and quality of life.

—Robert Anda, MD, MS, Co-Principal Investigator,
Adverse Childhood Experiences (ACE) Study

My task to survey the many complex, mind-body relationships was rendered much easier by the important contribution of Stockdale's review of resources and bibliographic references that complement this very interesting, easy-to-read, vignette-chock-full account. She combines humor and joy with serious scholarship in dealing with such severe diseases as cancer. This book is valuable to laypersons as well as to serious professionals in search of research-based information that is also fun to read.

–Luciano L'Abate, PhD, Professor Emeritus,
Georgia State University

This work offers tremendous insight into the lives of patients and their families dealing with life altering illness. I have seen this program turn an uphill, uncertain battle to one that empowers individuals and their families to believe that their journey will be a fulfilling and uplifting one.

—Gerry Goldklang, MD, Board Certifiied
Medical Oncologist, Georgia Cancer Specialists

As a primary care physician I have seen first-hand the tremendous effects of this program—from normalizing blood pressure and reversing insulin resistance and hyperglycemia, to improving adrenal function, chronic fatigue and other health problems. Patients reading this book not only become educated in the evidence behind behavioral medicine methods, they become inspired and empowered by scientifically based self-care strategies. As a result, it makes my day go by much better when seeing people who are able to be so proactive in their own healthcare. I recommend this book as a companion manual for better living, better health, and high-level wellness.

—Michael G. Milton, MD, MD-H,
Board Certified Family Physician

As a mind-body practitioner for over 20 years, I've always wished that I had one book to give to my patients that said it all in an easy-to-read format. It didn't exist, but now it does. Brenda's book is very enjoyable to read, and so specific that it gives readers a manual that they can use to feel empowered. Her protocol can actually help people learn to use their minds to heal their bodies before serious illnesses can take hold. For the skeptics, the science is all there and it's very compelling. For those already persuaded who want specific tools that they can use—they're here.

—Janet Eggan, MA, former clinical
director of Advanced Neuroscience

If you or someone you know has a chronic illness, or if you simply want to be your optimal self, *You Can Beat the Odds* is a must-read. Patients, clients, caregivers, and healthcare workers from many disciplines can immediately use the wisdom in this book, but because of Stockdale's accessible style, anyone would enjoy reading it. *You Can Beat the Odds* is full of rich scientific evidence balanced with anecdotal applications, practical exercises, and caring advice from one who knows first-hand the challenges of chronic illnesses.

—John F. Evans, PhD, Founder and Executive Director
of Wellness & Writing Connections

This book offers its readers a gentle but persuasive journey toward understanding the application of mind-body medicine. Ultimately, it represents a systematic lifestyle approach that complements the other primary health-determining factors, diet and exercise. Highly recommended.

—Robert Krikorian, PhD, Associate Professor of Psychiatry and Director, Cognitive Disorders Center, University of Cincinnati Academic Health Center

In *You Can Beat the Odds*, Brenda Stockdale provides for patients and family members the quintessential guidebook and companion towards healthy living and wellness. This book is not about concepts. It is about YOU. By incorporating personal experiences as well as real life stories about patients and individuals, she makes clear and practical the complex and current advances in the fields of epigenetics and psychoneuroimmunology. It is not merely about how these advances and studies can help you. It is the instruction book for ensuring that they do. For patients facing very challenging and grim diagnoses as well as individuals looking to enhance their overall well-being, mindfulness, and quality of life, *You Can Beat the Odds* is the long awaited manual on how to benefit immediately from this groundbreaking work. Now that science has met traditional practice, this is the required reading for anyone interested in learning these skills while understanding the evidence behind them.

—Chad A Levitt, MD, Board Certified Radiation Oncologist

Brenda Stockdale has taken the initial work of Carl Simonton, M.D., and Jeanne Achterberg to the next level of understanding and use for cancer patients. The clarity of explanation, scientific support, and completeness is remarkable. I personally loved the unique chapter on the healing power of music and sound. This increases the dimension of healing tools, and certainly reminds us of the universality of this dimension. In my opinion, this is the finest work presented on this critical subject of healing for cancer patients.

—Edward H. Gilbert, M.D., Radiation Oncologist, Medical Director, Simonton Center

You *Can* Beat the Odds

You *Can* Beat the Odds

Surprising Factors Behind Chronic Illness and Cancer

BRENDA STOCKDALE

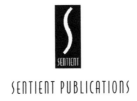

SENTIENT PUBLICATIONS

First Sentient Publications edition 2009
Copyright © 2009 by Brenda Stockdale

For permissions, see page 308.

A paperback original

Cover design by Kim Johansen, Black Dog Design
Book design by Timm Bryson

Library of Congress Cataloging-in-Publication Data
Stockdale, Brenda, [date]
 You can beat the odds : surprising factors behind chronic illness and
cancer / Brenda Stockdale.
     p. cm.
 Includes bibliographical references and index.
 ISBN 978-1-59181-079-7
 1. Stress management. 2. Medicine, Psychosomatic. 3. Chronic diseases.
4. Cancer. I. Title.
 RA785.S755 2009
 616.001'9--dc22

                         2009018765

Printed in the United States of America
10 9 8 7 6 5 4 3 2

SENTIENT PUBLICATIONS
A Limited Liability Company
1113 Spruce Street
Boulder, CO 80302
www.sentientpublications.com

CONTENTS

WEEK SIX

Dedicated to Robert Crouse Stockdale, who taught me the power of hope, the value of character and the wisdom in acknowledging that each day could be my last. This is for you, Dad.

In Loving Memory of Deirdre Davis Brigham.

A NOTE TO THE READER

Hundreds of research articles are cited in this work and many of the authors were generous with their time—patiently answering my questions and sharing their perspective. Any errors in translating their ideas or work are mine and mine alone. In addition to highlighting relevant research and science, this book documents people—the individuals behind the science—their personal stories and often remarkable recoveries. While the gist of their experience and medical details are correct, unless a first and last name is given, identifying characteristics have been altered. For privacy purposes every effort has been made to honor and protect their anonymity while holding true to medical accuracy. Names have been changed, events transposed, and occasionally, clinical stories merged in order to protect identity. As with any health book, establishing a solid healing partnership with a trusted physician is highly recommended. Use good common sense—never use anything in any book in the place of sound medical therapies and recommendations. Any suggestions or ideas presented in the book should only be used under the guidance of a physician, psychotherapist, or other health care provider and are not intended to treat any disease or condition or replace professional medical treatment. The author, publisher, and all others associated with this book cannot be held liable for any consequences of undertaking ideas or suggestions in this book whether or not under the care of a licensed professional.

FOREWORD BY BERNIE SIEGEL, M.D.

No one lives forever, so the odds of your becoming immortal are not too good whether you read this book or not. However, I have learned that there is a pattern of behavior which long term survivors and those who exceed expectations display that relates to their not dying when expected to. Individuals are not a statistic and their behavior, desire and intention play a significant role in their ability to beat the odds.

Decades ago psychologist Bruno Klopfer was able to predict correctly from personality profiles alone in nineteen out of twenty-four cases who would have a slow growing tumor and who would have a rapidly growing tumor. Early in this century psychologists wrote about this because they saw the role relationships and lifestyle play in the onset of disease. Monday morning is a good example. Your body loves you but if you do not love your life the physical problems and afflictions will increase dramatically. So Monday morning we have more suicides, strokes, heart attacks and illnesses.

Today studies are being done about things which decades ago no one studied because they didn't believe they could play a role in survival. I was criticized greatly for asking patients about what was going on in their lives. My words were misinterpreted as blaming the patient. I was trying to determine what made the individual vulnerable at a certain time.

Today studies reveal the benefits of laughter in the survival of cancer patients. How loneliness affects the genes which control immune function and how women live longer than men, and married men longer than single men, with the same cancers. It is not about female hormones protecting the women and the men who sleep with them but about relationships and connections and their role in survival. However, I also try to teach people to not live a role as I see women dying when the kids leave home and men getting sick when they can't work anymore.

Years ago psychologists and Jungian therapists saw cancer as growth gone wrong, a message to people to take a new road in their lives. Psychiatrist Karl Menninger told me he was going to write a book entitled *Twelve Hopeless Cases* about twelve people who were alive and well after being told they were all going to die. Why did they survive because of the changes they made in their lives? He also said to me after my book *Love, Medicine & Miracles* came out, "I don't have to write it because you have."

I saw this happen when I founded ECaP in 1978, when a patient of mine said to me, "I need to know how to live between office visits." To make a long story short I noticed when you helped people to live they didn't die when they were supposed to. They literally saved their lives by starting to live authentically, based upon what made them happy, and not just living the way the authorities in their life imposed upon them.

Mind and body are a unit. I learned about the use of dreams and spontaneous drawings in diagnosing and treating disease. Carl Jung interpreted a dream and correctly diagnosed a brain tumor. I have never met a medical student who has been told that. When people draw their treatment as the devil giving them poison or say they hate their doctor more than their cancer because doctors have made them bald, ugly and horrible, they have a problem with treatment and its side effects. The mind is a powerful thing and can kill or cure based upon what the person believes. Wordswordswords are hypnotic when they come from an authority and can become swords.

What I try to do, and this book helps us to understand, is to look at what our potential is and try to achieve it. What are we capable of is the question. When one is brought up with love and has self worth and self esteem one does not fear becoming a responsible participant in one's life rather than a submissive, suffering patient. So read on and put the information and inspiration together and the results will impress you as they did me many years ago.

BERNIE SIEGEL, M.D.
August, 2009

ॐ 1 ॐ

Launching Your Program
for Optimal Immunity

*Illness is the night-side of life, a more onerous citizenship.
Everyone who is born holds dual citizenship, in the kingdom
of the well and in the kingdom of the sick.*

—SUSAN SONTAG

"Houston, we have a problem." Those now famous words brought the plight of the three astronauts on Apollo 13 onto televisions and radios around the world and sparked a miracle of engineering teamwork that would bring those men home alive.

Although we'll never know most of their names, the best and the brightest minds were put to use that day to save the lives of the astronauts hurtling through space at thirty-five thousand miles per hour in a jury-rigged spacecraft. For the public, there were no faces for the legion of ground-bound engineers, just those of the men whose lives were at risk: Jim Lovell, Jack Swigert, and Fred Haise.

The historic flight had been uneventful until, halfway to the moon, an unexpected rumble was followed by crystallized particles floating in space. The astronauts knew then that the two oxygen tanks had ruptured and their air supply was falling, venting out into space, and their lives were in danger. The momentous success of the rescue mission would require a novel application of scientific principles and the collective wisdom of the experts on the ground.

The moon landings involved so many elements that had to perform perfectly together that hundreds of rocket scientists were required to determine the weakest links and strategize backup measures. My father was one of them. As he explains it to me, at the time of the crisis, experts in engineering and physical science worked together at a frantic pace to create a plan that would bring the astronauts back to earth. And in only eight hours they had one. Teams of brainy pencil pushers, working behind the scenes, were going to tell the men whose lives were at stake what they needed to do. The astronauts put their trust in these scientists and the plan was implemented. The lunar landing module had oxygen; the young men crawled into their new spaceship and used the gravity of the moon to slingshot them back to earth.

Most of the failures on the moon missions, as well as other complex missile systems, involved some of the simplest components—a wiring connection or a loose part—that might otherwise seem inconsequential. Like these spacecraft with so many fragile and sensitive parts, our own health and vitality can be upended by a single glitch in any one of a number of systems, and the smallest defect in the smallest part can yield hazardous results. Our physical bodies are far more complex than a missile or a spacecraft and healing can require miracle workers similar to those involved in that great and famous Apollo rescue mission. When fighting for your life or facing a challenging diagnosis, you deserve nothing less than the greatest minds working together on your behalf. Part chance, part science and design—not a piece of evidence can be overlooked—the great and the small must all come together in a remarkable way and in record time. It's a time when clear information and attention to detail offer distinct benefits (something you really want on your side when you're battling the odds, and when the colossal impact of all the possibilities cannot be underestimated).

This challenge demands a resource to guide us through turbulence and change, capitalizing on the teamwork of the best and the brightest, for a shortcut to beating the odds. In the six-week program outlined in this book, strategies from leaders in multiple disciplines help put the odds back on your side, so you can harness all the available technologies quickly and easily. Here, you can gain an advantage with up-to-the-minute information about a rapidly building body of discoveries that can enhance your healing potential on the deepest possible level. The program features life-changing discoveries by pioneering psychoneuroimmunoligists, epigeneticists, psychobiologists, scientists, physicians, medical researchers, epidemiologists, and stress researchers, among others.

The result is a compendium of practical and essential information for a lifelong program of what to do to stay strong. If you already enjoy great health, the program outlined here can help you keep it—you'll see that even small changes now can lead to a huge impact later. But if you are facing a health challenge, every piece of information makes a difference, as nothing can be left to chance or be overlooked.

Beyond Diet and Exercise

Aside from a general awareness of prevention through diet and exercise, current thinking in health care is changing in ways that are both startling and not generally understood by those outside of the research fields. The evidence is breathtaking. Technologies, skills, and behaviors—above and beyond diet and exercise—influence gene expression, hormone levels, bone density, blood pressure, and other processes once thought to be beyond our control. Crucial findings reveal that chemicals released in the emotional part of your brain (called the limbic system) attach directly to your white blood cells—the backbone of your immune system—in a lock and key fashion. This means that the way we think, feel, and behave has a direct effect on the way these cells operate—whether they swim rapidly and detect invader cells, go awry and attack healthy tissue, or become confused and allow unhealthy cells to proliferate. From brain to body and back again, the outcome of cell-to-cell communication is monumental: the result could be a healthy immune system, or if things go wrong, it could be the beginning of a malignant tumor or an autoimmune disease.

Nearly all aspects of our health and well-being are impacted by the momentous implications of these recent discoveries. For example, in the highly charged realms of genetics and microbiology, frontier science sparked the exciting new awareness that even our genetic inheritance is not as fixed as we may have thought. In fact, only 5 percent of cancer and cardiovascular patients can attribute their disease solely to heredity. Compelling new evidence shows we can even enhance our DNA!

While writing this book, I was asked to give a brief presentation about my work to a group of philanthropists. Afterwards, almost giddy with relief, a woman said, "Finally, a health book that's not about diet and exercise!" We all laughed. But while sound nutrition and exercise cannot be overlooked, new research shows there are other factors at play—risks greater than even smoking, obesity, or cholesterol—that are proven to increase mortality rates of virtually every disease.

Particularly persuasive are findings from a landmark study at the CDC (Centers for Disease Control) establishing that factors *other* than diet and exercise contribute the greatest risks associated with some of our biggest killers, including heart and lung disease. The peculiar difficulties encountered by the lead authors of the study shed light on why you may not know about their astonishing results. (You'll read more about this remarkable investigation in chapter 7.)

This new information hasn't intentionally been swept under the rug. In medical settings, time is often critical, making it extremely difficult to adequately address such issues, and as a result, the risk factors hover on the sidelines. This situation is gradually changing. For example, the program described in this book is provided at a cancer center and a primary care practice in Atlanta, while Harvard's medical centers, MD Anderson, and Memorial Sloan-Kettering, have similar programs for cancer and chronic disease.

As testament to the effectiveness and enormous cost-saving potential of programs like this, insurance companies have added codes for reimbursement of these new methods for treatment of heart disease, diabetes, autoimmunity, pain management, and overall wellness. Still other insurers offer discounted rates for individuals who complete programs similar to this one.[1] Even so, concerned physicians tell me that while the evidence is robust, these risk factors—and what to do about them—remain in the background. This book is a response, in part, to the challenge of bringing life-enhancing strategies into standard medical settings and into your life.

Myths and Medicine

As we begin this new century, newfangled interventions, genetic engineering, and smart cells are leading us into ground-breaking territory, ripe with promise. But what we do today can make or break our ability to participate and respond to these promises of tomorrow. To benefit, we can't afford to be side tracked by trends or complacent thinking. Real evidence is the key. Our universal quest for health and wellness—and accurate information—is an ancient one. As evidenced by the two thousand Egyptian prescriptions recorded on papyri and the first pharmacopoeia, *De Materia Medica*, compiled in 50 AD, people have long searched for an edge to beating the odds. The historical record demonstrates some recommendations were more effective than others—applying beetle dung to a wound may not have helped much, but the medicinal value of foxglove was later found to be a true tonic for people with heart conditions and is now prescribed as digitalis. The laws of the Israelites recorded in the Bible—such as hand washing, and quarantining the ill and the dead—had to be rediscovered in the nineteenth century before their implementation could save lives in the western world. But just because a treatment enjoyed popularity didn't mean it had merit—bloodletting, with leeches or knives, was an undisputed remedy for nearly any ailment for more than a millennium, reaching its peak at the beginning of the nineteenth century, and finally dying out (forgive the irony) by that century's end.

In science, nearly everything is provisional. It wasn't all that long ago that the appendix was believed to be vestigial, or basically useless, but now we know it's actually a component of the immune system in the gut. Until recently, lupus, chronic fatigue, Hashimoto's disease, hypertension, heart disease, and cancer were not thought to be related, but considered separate entities operating under their own banner, as it were. But cutting edge science reveals that these diseases share a common origin—chronic inflammation[2]—and the pharmaceutical giants of the world have their financial resources aimed sharply at this linchpin.

The brutal impact of this single trigger, chronic inflammation, is astounding in the numbers affected: over one hundred twenty-eight million people. Of those, according to the World Health Organization, nearly seventeen million people around the globe die each year of cardiovascular disease, while another twenty million survive, but deal with the aftermath of heart attacks and strokes. They join ten million others who are cancer survivors. But it doesn't stop there: In the United States alone, over twenty million people currently have diabetes, while another fifty-four million have prediabetes, and over eight million are managing an autoimmune disease at any given time. This new way of thinking about how we stay healthy—and how we get sick—can affect how we approach almost any illness or condition.

The Crucible

As with any rescue mission, whether it's from space, a burning building, or a threatening diagnosis, the heroes are the ones whose lives are on the line, and a remarkable outcome requires determination and imagination from all the players. When I first met Frank Hawkins, he told me that he hadn't been particularly concerned when he experienced a mysterious pain in his side and a bit of indigestion. But despite being treated for ulcers, the discomfort didn't entirely disappear and eventually intense back pain on a business trip stopped him in his tracks. Returning home from Florida, his wife teased him about his great tan. As it turned out, he wasn't tan, but was jaundiced. Exploratory surgery revealed pancreatic cancer too far advanced for treatment of any kind. When Frank asked about his options the doctor replied that there weren't any. "We'll make it as easy on you as we can but you need to just go home and get your affairs in order," adding that Frank had a few weeks to live—maybe six, maybe more.

Frank determined then that no one person was going to dictate the outcome and gave himself options that the doctor had denied. Frank explains, "After I picked myself up off the floor I went back to my original physician and asked for a referral to another cancer specialist." So, along with his wife, Sarah, Frank consulted medical oncologist Gerald Goldklang, M.D., who spoke about perspectives like "will to live" and "fighting spirit." Formerly fuzzy concepts like these have made their way into laboratories and research projects around the globe, and while much remains mysterious about their effects, Frank was convinced that Dr. Goldklang would champion and support him in his fight for life— regardless of the outcome. As Frank puts it, "I wasn't going down without a struggle." Along with offering a new chemotherapy, Dr. Goldklang recommended that Frank and Sarah attend my six-week program (which meets once a week) at the cancer center.

Like the Apollo 13 astronauts, from the crucible of diagnosis, Frank had little to lose. Although fatigued, he began chemotherapy and attended his first class with me the following week. I was stunned at his jaundice and pallor. Yet despite losing an astonishing amount of weight, he continued with his medical treatment, his job, and the activities that he and Sarah loved—spending time in the mountains, gardening, attending street-rod car shows and craft exhibits. Four weeks went by, then six, then eight—each week becoming a celebratory milestone. A few months later scans revealed that the chemotherapy had greatly reduced the size of the tumor and an innovative surgical procedure was cautiously offered. The surgeon met with Frank and openly shared his concern. He had only performed one other procedure like it and the results were not good. But Frank was willing to try. As he recovered from the operation, just six months after being told to get his affairs in order, the specialist walked into the room and pronounced Frank cancer free. More than eleven years later, that is still the case. Recently Frank and Sarah dropped in on one of our classes just to say hello. While there is no standard cure for pancreatic cancer, the science behind that story is both eye-opening and practical. What you are about to read shows you how to use that science to your great advantage in everyday life.

Personalizing Your Program: How It Works

But life is complicated, and dealing with a chronic, life-challenging illness makes it more so. With our busy lives, we need strong reasons and compelling evidence to make the effort to learn something new. My goal in writing this book is to streamline that process. With research in science and medicine on your side, and backed by a solid relationship with your medical team, you can quickly take advantage of life-enhancing thinking. Designed to complement a busy lifestyle, each component works in tandem with the rest, as research-based skills and techniques allow you to take charge of your health in new and powerful ways.

> *Hope is definitely not the same thing as optimism.*
> *It is not the conviction that something will turn out well,*
> *but the certainty that something makes sense, regardless of how it turns out.*
>
> —VACLAV HAVEL, WRITER
> AND PRESIDENT OF THE
> CZECH REPUBLIC

Book chapters are grouped into individual weeks of the six-week program. (For example, chapters 2 and 3 are covered in week two of the program and so on.) Flush with evidence, the science behind each concept is presented clearly under the *How We Know* headings so you'll understand what that particular technique or technology can do for you. A no-nonsense approach delivers the research in an easy-to-understand way so you can see how these methods are linked with improved outcomes and positive whole-body effects. Taken from over a decade of feedback, many practical examples of how others have used these strategies are included. And each week in the program you'll meet a physician, scientist, or other medical professional who has personally used that concept in his or her own life. If you'd like more information on a particular topic, the *Resource Guide* at the back of the book can help.

Under the headings *Get Started Now,* you'll see material that tells you how to put the research into action so you can begin using it right away. Here, interactive features such as quizzes, website questionnaires, and worksheets help you integrate the new insights you've gained so you can personalize your program and jump-start your healing potential. There may be more *Get Started Now* exercises than you can do in one week, so you can treat them like handouts and set some aside for later. For example, in the very first week of the program you will discover how the chemicals in your mind affect not only your immune system, but also all the glands and hormones of your body, including your intestines and the lining of your blood vessels. You'll find out how you might (unknowingly) be working against yourself and you'll be given a simple technique to reduce inflammation and protect your brain, bones, blood pressure, gut, and genes.

Subsequent chapters bring you up to speed, progressively revealing hidden risk factors and how you can combat them with proven research-based strategies that enhance our health and well-being. You may choose to read all the way through the book and then go back and spend a week reflecting on a particular aspect of the program. There are no rules for moving through the book but the research is presented progressively, so it will make more sense if you review it in the order given. As each chapter builds upon the knowledge of the last, you'll gain momentum exponentially as every action, no matter how small, has an effect. Whether learning how to use sound as medicine, reduce damaging stress hormones, or tip the scales of genetic expression in your favor, you'll find an abundance of self-care strategies to choose from or combine, along with plenty of practical suggestions, reliable research, and powerful stories that provide a personal side to the science.

Stacking the Deck

I often say I teach what I need to know. I was twenty-one when I lost the feeling in my feet. At the time I thought it was temporary and just switched to shoes that I wouldn't slip out of. Odd flashes of light at the periphery of my sight and other visual distortions I couldn't ignore sent me to my physician; and when I lost sensation on one side of my body, I was referred to a neurologist. After a lumbar puncture, scans, an MRI, and loads of blood work, I was sent home with a diagnosis of multiple sclerosis.

On the whole I did quite well, but kidney infections—and later lung infections—became so chronic that as a preventive measure, I was prescribed a maintenance antibiotic that I took every day for five years. About that time, routine blood work came back looking suspiciously like scleroderma and I was sent to another specialist who wanted to tack that on top of the diagnosis of MS. Frustrated and more than a little freaked out, I felt it was a good time for an evaluation by the team approach at the Mayo Clinic. There, specialists diagnosed that I had neither MS nor scleroderma, but systemic lupus erythematosus (SLE) all along. As I read up on this new condition I happened upon an emerging field of study called psychoneuroimmunology, or PNI for short. This compelling science takes a close look at the foundations of disease, and specifically, how chemicals in our mind impact our immune system.

I was intrigued. With kidney and central nervous system impairment, I had little to lose. Immersing myself in research and connecting with expert guidance, my physician at the Mayo Clinic, Scott Percellin, M.D., provided careful monitoring and support as I applied what I was learning to my own life. (For details see the Acknowledgements.) Shortly thereafter, as the clinical assistant to the national PNI (psychoneuroimmunology) program Getting Well, I witnessed firsthand how certain skills and behaviors could alter or heal physical processes.

Remarkable recoveries met me every step of the way and I learned to respect that while principles were at play, there was no one *right* way to heal. Men and women from teenagers to seniors employed these modalities in their own unique and very individual ways and experienced benefits. When the feeling in my feet returned, I knew I was on to something. A few months later I was off antibiotics completely—and I've not had a kidney or lung infection since. The result has been a clinical and serological remission that has lasted over fifteen years. (At times I've been a remedial student, so fortunately or unfortunately, I've had other reminders to practice what I preach!)

The science behind the rescue mission of Apollo 13 wasn't new but it was clever. The teams of experts used available knowledge and applied it in a remarkable way to an unprecedented situation for a near miraculous result. In the same way, some of what helped Frank and me wasn't necessarily new, but the application was novel to us. Over the last decade, though, exciting new discoveries have come to light. The next chapter opens the door to recent findings that shed light on recoveries like ours.

Since my own healing experience, I have witnessed many "miracles" even more profound. The heroes of the book—the everyday people whose lives are on the line—furnish faces for the mystery and majesty of remarkable recovery, bring to life its research and theories, and lend substance to statistics with stories that resonate with all who wish to beat the odds. I hope that you may be as inspired by the indomitable spirit, courage, and strength of will of these heroes as I have been. Unless otherwise indicated, I know these people personally and although most of their identities are cloaked, the medical specifics and what they did about their health challenges are all very real. (As a key, when a last name is listed, as in Frank's case, the identity is intact and unaltered.)

Getting Well

The seeds for this six-week program began while I was working at Getting Well, the PNI program mentioned above, in Orlando, Florida. Participating required a residential stay of ten days to one month and so was out of reach for some patients. Working with busy people, it became important to me to design a how-to program, linking expert guidance with strategies proven to positively influence health for maximum effect in the shortest possible time. Later, as the program director for Yale surgeon Bernie Siegel's Exceptional Cancer Patients' (ECaP) organization in Connecticut, I had the opportunity to put the program into play and bring it to life. It was accepted by the president at the time of the American Cancer Society and the chief oncologist of the Helen and Harry Gray Cancer Center, Dr. Andrew Salner, a compassionate and caring physician, dedicated to bringing all possible tools together for the optimal advantage of the tens of thousands who walk through the center's doors each year.

After relocating to the southeast, I happened upon an article in *Atlanta Magazine* about a cancer specialist, Dr. Gerry Goldklang. I thought to myself that if I were ever to work with a local oncologist, he would be the one. At the time, Tim Albaitis—my co-director at ECaP—and I were putting together weeklong educational programs for folks with chronic illness or cancer. People flew in from all over the world to participate. We had a group (as you can tell, I'm big into the team approach) of wonderful professionals, each with a different specialty and perspective, and had a great time working together. But when it came time to focus closer to home, I called Dr. Goldklang and we set up a time to meet. As it happened, Dr. Goldklang had just returned from an international conference where this new evidence was presented and he was committed to providing it for patients and the community. And so it began.

Soon this program was introduced to a primary care practice where those with autoimmunity, diabetes, high blood pressure, and other conditions could apply the research to their advantage as well. As you will see, the techniques and strategies for health and wellness you're about to discover are not meant to replace your medical protocol but to enhance it, working hand-in-glove with whatever treatment modality you've chosen. Applying expert guidance and rallying your ability to heal from within, whether you are using conventional or complementary medicine, or both, will help you gain the most from any treatment. Like the astronauts of Apollo 13 who became instrumental in their own rescue mission, taking personal responsibility for our health enhances the outcome. The aspects of the program have a cumulative effect, and the combinations can tip the odds in your favor. Perhaps most importantly, the program's solid scientific base complements a variety of worldviews.

As one woman put it, patients benefit and doctors appreciate it. But after attending the program, people wanted something to refer to and were overwhelmed by the many titles on my suggested reading list. They repeatedly requested a book based on the program. While no one book can offer the definitive word on wellness, my goal was to provide a blueprint of the references that have inspired others and me, along with a practical guide to applying the principles in everyday life. With thanks to the persistence of patients and professionals who have helped me along the way, I offer the result of all these combined efforts, which you now hold in your hands.

The Number Nine Bus

Life is nothing if not unpredictable. In a post 9/11 world of color-coded anxiety, we need real help for real problems and coping strategies for even scarier imagined ones. Whether through a life-challenging diagnosis or rapidly changing world events, we are reminded that we live daily with uncertainty—and always have. People who do all the right things can die far too young, while others, who perhaps seem just too mean, may do all the wrong things and outlive everybody.

This truth wasn't lost on Joe Kogel. When I was at Getting Well, Joe spoke to a packed auditorium about his diagnosis of metastatic melanoma (a deadly type of skin cancer that had spread) and used a metaphor I've never forgotten. Like Frank, his prognosis was grim and he didn't know anybody personally who had beaten the particular odds he faced, but that wasn't a drawback for Joe. He said we could all wake up tomorrow and hear that a cure for cancer or heart disease had been discovered, but there's still the number nine bus taking us out on a harmless Thursday afternoon. I've used this metaphor for years and one day a patient asked what my last thoughts would be if I ever saw the number nine bus bearing down on me in the middle of a busy intersection. "It was only supposed to be a metaphor!" was my response. Of course, one day we'll each meet our own metaphor, so to speak, but until then we keep looking both ways when we cross the street. It doesn't guarantee us safe passage but it definitely increases our odds. By the way, eighteen years later Joe is still cancer free.

The tools, techniques, and methods you'll discover here serve as a complement to your own intuitive wisdom and the knowledge and skills you have already accumulated. In combination they shape and bring to life your own personal program of wellness and assist you in making the most of this time of crisis and change. It is my wish that the information and strategies contained in these six weeks serve as a road map on your journey to optimal health and leave you feeling empowered for whatever the future may bring.

Week One

The Biology of Miracles:
The Science Behind Beating the Odds

The human body is its own best apothecary because the most successful prescriptions are those that are filled by the body itself.

—NORMAN COUSINS

Nicholas Hall, Ph.D., a researcher in psychoneuroimmunology (or PNI), doesn't need a cheap trick to hold anybody's attention. Attractive, charming, and articulate, his lectures are so engaging that the science he's presenting becomes almost indistinguishable from the stories they revolve around. Since he put himself through college by wrestling alligators and milking rattlesnakes, and willingly participated in what has been called the most dangerous boat race in the world, he certainly has a lot of material to choose from. But instead, he introduces his presentations by reading a spicy excerpt from *Lady Chatterley's Lover.* He notes that the steamy passage makes the audience very much aware that the mind influences the body!

While we're not going there, think for a moment about your favorite food. Close your eyes. Imagine the aroma, the texture, and the taste.

Do you salivate? Now imagine biting into a juicy, sour lemon. What happens? Perhaps you can recall a time when someone told you an awesome story and the hair on your arms stood on end. In that very instant, your hair follicles responded to a story you heard. What happens when you blush? Your capillaries open wide rapidly—to something someone said or did—and the blood rushes to your face.

Your Brain as a Pharmacy

These are palpable and visible reactions your body has to images, thoughts, and words. These responses range from the ordinary, like salivating, to the offbeat, like rashes, that come and go depending on a person's state of mind. On a cellular level, this communication is occurring between mind and body throughout the day. Your brain is like a virtual pharmacy, influencing your body as it responds to your emotions and to your thinking processes. In every moment of our lives, an ever-changing array of hormones and molecules interact, nudging us either toward health or toward disease. You already dip into this infinite apothecary on a regular basis, whether or not you are aware of it.

Technical advances today allow us to peer into some emotional states, mapping and measuring dozens of chemical correlates to the way we think and feel that help or hinder our immune system. Since 1974, when Professor of Psychosocial Medicine Robert Ader, M.D., first demonstrated that rats could be conditioned to influence their immune system, studies have expanded and become more sophisticated, using emotional states, perceptions, and thoughts, instead of only physical or chemical substances, as the conditioning stimuli.[3] For example, students viewing a film of Mother Teresa showed an increase in immunoglobulin-A in their saliva, which is a positive immune influence.[4] (By the way, this held true for even those students who didn't like Mother Teresa.) Correspondingly, Nazi film footage decreased the immune response of students.

Multiple experiments conducted by Professor Christian Keysers of the Social Brain Laboratory show that simply observing an activity stimulates the same part of the brain as if you were personally participating.[5] In one experiment when subjects watched a video in which an actor's legs were brushed with a glove, the exact same part of their brain "lit up" as if their own legs had been brushed. In another (if you can handle the *ewww* factor) watching a video of someone repulsed by a smell stimulated an identical area of the brain in subjects who had been exposed to actual rotting food and other nauseating scents.

In either case, how we think, the stories we tell ourselves, and the images we hold in our mind generate a biological effect that enables us to examine the molecular basis of emotion. That effect begins in a tiny part of the brain called the limbic system. This is where your experience is translated into a physical reality—like when your heart races because you are scared or excited. In this magical area of the brain sights, sounds, thoughts, and feelings are translated into biological events at lightning speed. The physical changes I've mentioned are ones you can see and feel, but most occur silently and invisibly throughout the day whether or not you are aware of them.

When the Body Says No

A physician examined a woman with widespread metastatic cancer and found that the cancer had suddenly regressed to the point that she was in fact completely cancer-free.[6] What had happened? An otherwise dry medical abstract reads, "A much hated husband dropped dead." What this case so dramatically attests to, aside from the perils of matrimonial contempt, is a phenomenon known as spontaneous remission. Consider the following two accounts closer to home—one from the primary care practice where I work and one from Getting Well.

> *Learn your theories as well as you can, but put them aside when you touch the miracle of the living soul.*
>
> —CARL JUNG

The young physician thought he had made a mistake. He tapped Jill's tendon to trigger the reflex again, and the tendon responded with alacrity, arching and descending rapidly. Just a few weeks ago, it had been slow and sluggish. This simple reflex test measures the body's use of thyroid hormone.[7] Blood work indicated that Jill didn't have a simple case of hypothyroidism, but an autoimmune variety called Hashimoto's. If the reflex is slow and non-responsive, it is technically impossible to alter its function without supplementing thyroid hormone. But Jill had taken none. However, she had been practicing the tools she learned in this program and was beginning to see results. Curious, the physician ordered labs that confirmed her Hashimoto's was in remission.

Mark was told that his rare form of salivary gland cancer had been successfully and completely removed and there was no need to worry about a recurrence. But, three years later, while sitting on the beach in Plum Island, Massachusetts, he intuitively reached up, touched his jaw and felt the growth again. This time there were no smooth assurances. The cancer had metastasized (or spread) and the specialists levied their sentence: with surgery, radiation, and chemotherapy, he had, at best, six months to live. The surgery itself would sever the facial nerve, leaving him scarred and unable to smile for the remaining months of his life.

Devastated, he left the hospital, got into his car and drove, and drove, and drove. While driving he heard something on the radio about a program called Getting Well, in Orlando, Florida. He decided he had little to lose. He scheduled his flight and arrived in Orlando, shell-shocked but open-minded. Mark continued to practice what he had learned at Getting Well after he returned home, and in a stroke of salvation, Mark was pronounced cancer-free three months later. Fifteen years later, that is still the case, and Mark is living proof of a miracle recovery.

No one can say that they have a cure for cancer or autoimmune disease. In medical jargon, recoveries like that of Frank Hawkins, whom you met in chapter 1, and the two cases just cited, are spoken of as "spontaneous remissions," which is not meant to imply that it occurs suddenly, but that the remission or regression has no known explanation. The self-healing generated by Frank, Jill, and Mark, while perhaps rare, are by no means isolated occurrences. The Remission Project of the Institute of Noetic Sciences (IONS) has assembled the largest database of medically reported cases of spontaneous remission in the world. Appropriately entitled *Spontaneous Remission*,[8] it contains thousands of medically documented cases of people who beat the odds, with diseases ranging from Hashimoto's to Kaposi's sarcoma and HIV to bone cancer. As vast as this documentation is, none of the men and women that I have met personally are included in the volume and likely none of the folks that you know are either. (Imagine how large the database might really be if everyone were counted!)

Gloomy prognostications though, like Frank's and Mark's, can be uncannily powerful. As a stopgap against such fatalism and as a distinct and solid reminder of possibilities, I keep a copy of this large volume of hope at the cancer center and in the primary care practice where I work. (The database is now available online; see the Resource Guide for more information.) Cases like these show that there is much more to getting well or getting sick than genetics, and much more to survival than prognostics. These documented recoveries seem linked to a spectacular switch, a skeleton key of genetic expression.

The Genie in Your Genes

It wasn't a trickle but a cascade of discoveries that toppled the idea that genes control our destiny.[9] When the Human Genome project began in 1990, researchers were confident it would offer up all the secrets of who gets sick and why, and hopes for long-sought cures for terrible diseases were pinned to the project. Scientists assumed that the difference in complexity between ourselves and lower life forms, such as insects and worms, would be explained by the number of our genes. A fruit fly, for instance, has about fifteen thousand genes, a common worm twenty-four thousand. In contrast, the human body was expected to have over a hundred thousand genes. When the fifteen-year project was concluded, researchers were astonished to discover that we have about the same number of genes as a worm or a rodent. (I know what you're thinking, and well, I was too, but this is serious research—not a time to be recasting your least favorite people as worms or rats!) All joking aside, it became clear that the number of genes couldn't possibly account for the differences between humans and worms.

The meaning behind the genes you carry was further questioned when it was discovered that having the gene that predisposes you to a particular disease doesn't mean that you will actually get the disease. This might be comforting if you've been tempted to undergo genetic testing, which can be intimidating. When I personally underwent genetic testing for a project I was curious about, the number of scary genes I had inherited was staggering. But, like everyone else, I've only manifested a certain sequence of those unhealthy genes I carry, not all of them.

These limitations, though, haven't discouraged frontier labs from springing up, promising to unlock the secrets of your DNA—from character traits to your personal risk of developing a host of awful diseases. Medical geneticist Dr. Wylie Burke and H. Gilbert Welch, an internist and professor at Dartmouth, warn that while these labs tap into our desire for control the information is not as good as we might think. "This may be a novel hook, but it's really pretty frivolous stuff...[and their advice is to] save your money, and spare your health."[10]

A case in point: When Robert Green, a medical researcher in Boston, Massachusetts, was offered complimentary genetic screening by a leading laboratory, he was curious to see if he had the ApoE gene, which can indicate a potential risk of Alzheimer's disease. It was the very condition he had been researching for a decade, and he was relieved to find his risk was quite low. Yet the report also disclosed that Robert had only an average risk of heart disease, when just the year before, at fifty-two, he had a triple bypass due to coronary artery disease. He doesn't smoke, is not overweight, exercises, and has normal cholesterol levels. Traditional thinking would have us believe that his risk is entirely genetic—yet no great risk was revealed by the screening.[11]

Bruce Lipton, cellular biologist and genetic pioneer of Stanford University and the University of Wisconsin's School of Medicine, agrees with Burke and Welch on the limited value of genetic testing, explaining that everything we think and do—what we eat, how we feel, how we respond to stress, and the toxins in our environment—affects our genetics.[12] These discoveries led to the newest player on the block, epigenetics, which literally means, "control above genetics." Making disease far more enigmatic, the area of epigenetics is a hotbed of research in widely diverse fields of science and medicine showing that, in addition to things like hazardous chemicals or nutrition, social and psychological factors also modulate or alter gene expression.

It's not that our genes themselves change; it's the way that they're expressed. While our DNA inherited from our parents is fixed, those genes have a special coating that acts like an antenna that scans the environment and translates what it finds into proteins that regulate our genes. That environment includes not only diet and exposure to toxins, but also our thoughts, our lifestyle, and even the way we were treated in early life. All of these factors are potent immune and genetic modulators. Even job stress and depression are linked to DNA damage. So the environment is key, controlling how and when a gene is expressed—turning them on or off as it were, with stunning results. You may have noticed this phenomenon in identical twins. Although they have exactly the same DNA over time, they can develop different appearances and even different diseases. While some scientists refer to a switching mechanism, turning genes on and off, Dr. Lipton explains that genes are actually uncovered—like a sleeve that fits over your arm—and healing, spontaneous or otherwise, results from re-covering (or covering over) that information. He likens our genetic inheritance to a drawer containing architectural plans. Having a few building designs tucked away in a drawer will never produce a building—for the building to come to life, someone has to take out a design plan, read it, and contract builders to produce it. Likewise, our genetic inheritance is hidden away, covered over, unless something happens to expose it and bring it to life.

There is no one-size-fits-all answer to any disease, no "all access pass" that shuttles you into a one-way diagnosis. As you learned in chapter 1, recent research indicates that only 5 percent of cancer and cardiovascular patients can attribute their diagnosis solely to heredity. Heart disease, diabetes, and cancer are not the result of carrying a single gene, but require the interaction between many genes and other factors too, such as emotions, the environment, and behavioral choices. So possessing a gene can be a relatively minor part of the equation. And even then, tantalizing research shows that once a gene is turned on, under the right circumstances it can be turned off. For example, using sensitive genomic analyses, Herbert Benson, associate professor of medicine at Harvard Medical School, recently discovered that harmful genes—leading to inflammation and free radical activity—could be neutralized by a regular relaxation practice.[13] Put simply, genes do not control our destiny.

Dr. Barry Bittman, neurologist and medical director of the Meadville Medical Center and ECaP, took the time to talk with me about his own genomic research. In his experiments, they examined forty-seven different genes associated with diabetes, cancer, heart disease, and inflammatory disorders. He found that when subjects are stressed, the genes that are turned on or exposed vary from person to person. While all cells contain the complete genome (except for mature red blood cells), they each have a unique expression, like a fingerprint. He explained that if thirty-two people had heart disease, all thirty-two would have a unique molecular response to stress, known as a stress signature. Bittman's studies, among a host of others, show that once genes are turned on or exposed, they can also be reversed (or covered over). Although gene therapy holds great promise, our genetic response to stress is deeply personal, as is the repair process.

Turning on and off harmful genes, however, doesn't necessarily involve cutting edge science. While strides in technology offer distinct advantages, much of what prevents disease lies in the interior of our hearts and minds. In a way, though, even this can be measured. Technology reveals that two great fatigue fighters (namely fascination and purpose) can cause our white blood cells, the fundamental structure of our immunity, to quicken and strike out against invaders, eliminating cancer or other harmful cells before they multiply. Internationally renowned psychobiologist Dr. Ernest Rossi writes that deeply meaningful experiences that incorporate "fascination, mysteriousness and tremendousness," signal "an unusually strong occurrence of gene expression, brain plasticity (more about this to come) and mind/body healing."[14]

Other mind-body and epigenetic interactions play out in less subtle ways. The loss of that sense of mystery and connectedness can sometimes extinguish, suddenly and unexpectedly, the breath or spark of life (ru'ach in Hebrew) that binds by invisible threads the pulsing rhythm of our cells and the breath in our lungs with the vast intentions of the heart. One of my close friends lost his mother to breast cancer. She had been quietly ill for quite some time and her passing, while intensely mourned, was not a shock. But his father's subsequent and sudden decline was. Like a bolt from the blue, after near-perfect health during a half-century of marriage, this strong and kindly man slipped silently into a coma and died a few weeks later.

Not long ago, cases like this were relegated to the nether world of anecdotal evidence, creating confusion and an uncomfortable climate for clinicians. Often, though, there is a collective truth in the stories we gather as a culture and as a people. My friend's story and others like it are now echoed and supported by hard and fast laboratory evidence that reveals low levels of lymphocyte activity (an essential part of immunity) occurring in men during the first few months of losing a spouse.[15]

The pharmacy in your mind is a major player in the game of genetic expression. This was lost on the ancient Egyptians who, while prizing the heart, considered the brain so unimportant that they discarded it when mummifying bodies. Progress was made two thousand years later when Hippocrates defied local tradition and labeled epilepsy a disorder of the brain rather than a curse from the gods. Presently, at Emory University, paralyzed patients are being taught how to control a computer by simply thinking about it. The cursor on the computer is moved according to the person's intent by electrical impulses from their brains.[16] But what does this mean in terms of immune function and survival? Quite a bit actually.

The Biology of Belief

In Italy, at the crossroads between the Alps and Lombardy, lies the University of Turin.[17] Its six-hundred-year history has seen the rise and fall of empires, as well as many plagues, famines, and wars, but today in the department of neuropsychiatry, experiments in pain control are taking place. In a recent study, Dr. Fabrizio Benedetti induced pain in subjects for several days and used morphine to keep the pain under control. Then on the last day of the experiment the morphine was withdrawn and instead a saline (salt) solution was given. The result? The saline solution worked just as well as the morphine.[18]

No doubt you are familiar with this response, called the placebo effect. But Dr. Benedetti took it a step further and added a morphine-blocking drug called naloxone and the pain returned. The pain-relieving power of the saline solution disappeared after the subjects received a drug to block morphine. Think for a moment about the implications: the saline (or placebo) stimulated the body to manufacture its own morphine, which was then blocked by the naloxone! Taken from the Latin, placebo or "if you please," has such a profound effect that every pharmaceutical and over-the-counter drug is tested against it as a touchstone. The effect is so significant that some drugs that make it into your medicine cabinet have been proven only slightly more effective than a placebo.

No less mind-bending are Benedetti's experiments with the mother of all anti-anxiety medication: Valium (diazepam). Sold on the street for serious dollars and wrangled out of reluctant physicians, Valium can pull you off the ceiling and bring you quietly back to center without a care in your trouble-riddled mind. I tried a similar medication myself once in preparation for a medical procedure. A few hours later I was at Home Depot's Expo Design Center laughing with strangers and helping them pick out their stuff. Whoa! I was social! The next day I asked my husband what our new sink was doing in the dining room. He raised his eyebrows saying I insisted he put it there after I made him hold it up over our existing sink (reasons unknown). Aside from a vague recollection of being very friendly to strangers I have no memory of any of this. (That's when I discovered that this class of drug, benzodiazepines, can have amnesiac effects; it's worth mentioning that they're also highly addictive.)

Given my response, imagine my surprise when Benedetti's research showed that diazepam doesn't work in patients after surgery unless they know they are taking it! (So if I had been told I was taking an aspirin would the sink have been in the garage rather than the dining room?) As it turns out, the drug's effectiveness depends on the placebo effect. Even for drugs that are effective apart from our expectations, the intensity of the results can be influenced by what we expect. Research shows that if people don't know that they are getting morphine, it requires a much higher dose to get the same effect as when they are aware of it being given.[19]

These mind boggling experiments upend our notions about evidence-based medicine. Can this be completely explained with what we currently know about biochemistry? No. But what we do know raises many interesting possibilities. The choices we make and the interpretations we assign events influence physiological outcomes. How our thoughts become molecules is an enigma; nevertheless, these electrical signals travel down neurons and cause a release of chemical messengers (known as neurotransmitters and neuropeptides). These messenger molecules are released into the bloodstream and into synapses (the connections between brain cells). They can also travel around the body and interact with other cells.

Here is the kicker: Chemical messengers released from the emotional center of your brain actually connect, in a true lock-and-key fashion, to receptor sites, or openings, on certain types of white blood cells. These critical cells are the backbone of your immune system, protecting you not only from cancer cells and viral invaders, but also modulating inflammation, the root cause in a multiplicity of disorders. Neuroscientist Candace Pert, who served as Chief of the Section on Brain Biochemistry of the Clinical Neuroscience Branch of the National Institute of Mental Health (NIMH), has shown that the interior grooves of each "door lock" on your microscopic white blood cells is precisely designed to receive a specific neuropeptide "key" from the emotional center of your brain. Imagine! From moment to moment how you think and feel releases a cascade of chemicals that lock into your immune cells. And that microscopic white blood cell has not just one or two different receptors for brain chemicals, but contains receptors for every neuropeptide discovered to date—about seventy so far. Pert estimates there may be over three hundred!

The part of your brain involved in regulating moods and feelings, the limbic system, is particularly rich in secreting these key-shaped molecules (neuropeptides). This means that our immune cells, among others, are constantly receiving messages sent by our brain and nervous system. (I've joked that my life would be easier if my immune system were more influenced by the logical and linear part of my brain rather than the emotional part!) But it goes both ways. Immune cells not only have receptors for various neuropeptides, they even manufacture their own. Some of these are actually brain chemicals. Since brain cells make immune chemicals and immune cells make brain chemicals, the road between mind and body is not a one-way street. A sensory drama unfolds as this interchange takes place throughout the various tissues and cells of body and brain, including our endocrine and circulatory systems. The upshot is that molecules interact on a moment-to-moment basis in a dynamic web, creating subtle and not-so-subtle shifts in our biology. (Consider what we know about babies in neonatal intensive care units, where touch stimulates the genes for growth!)

Your Gut Instinct

Given the fact that most of the chemicals in our minds have receptor sites (or links) throughout our tissues—the lining of our gut, our circulatory system, and our immune system—body and mind can no longer be subdivided. Every single nerve in our body and brain is modulated by messenger molecules—the ultimate common denominator, according to Pert, of all communication between mind, emotions, and behavior. We may think in terms of a nervous system or the immune system or hormones, but they are all part of a single supersystem that is so interrelated that some clinicians and researchers no longer refer to mind-body communication, but mind-body unity. It appears that the entire body is engineered as a "conversation," with each organ, tissue, cell, and gene speaking to the whole and back again. Even your stomach participates in the on-going dialogue.

Have you ever had a sensation that you described as a gut feeling? You may be surprised to know that it's not just a metaphor, but that the lining of your intestines is one of the richest receptor sites for brain chemicals in the human body. No organ system next to the brain has more nerve tissue than our gut, prompting scientists to refer to it as our "second brain." So the fabled gut instinct is actually an elegant example of mind-body communication. With this evidence in mind, we want to maintain a healthy respect for the messages coming from our bodies—it's not mind over matter—but mind and matter affecting each other. That is one reason why throughout this book you will find an emphasis on paying attention to how you feel, as that feeling represents a physiological event. We'll talk about using this intuitive awareness to your advantage (and how to enhance it) later, but for now give yourself permission to begin coaxing out this awareness by tuning in to how you feel about everyday things, such as what you want to wear or what you'll eat for lunch.

The Tipping Point

Like for Frank Hawkins, who beat pancreatic cancer, and my friend's father, who suddenly declined after his wife's death, the factors that most impact your health are not so much the genes that you've inherited, but instead are more the moment-by-moment expression of those genes. Epigenetics are influenced by a multiplicity of factors, not the least of which is stress. In recent years, stress has been linked to every major cause of death. Scientific literature is packed with research from medicine, neuroscience, and genetics showing that stress wreaks havoc with your entire system, altering gene expression and making you more susceptible to just about everything, from gum disease to a heart attack.

In fact, the effect of your emotional state on your cells is so perfectly attuned that the likelihood of catching a cold virus can be predicted based on that state. Think about how often you've heard someone in the middle of a difficult situation, such as a rancorous divorce or a lay-off from work, blame it on stress when they come down with a virus or the flu. And now you know why: investigators have discovered nerve cells that communicate directly with your brain and other organs that are vital to immunity, such as the spleen and the thymus (once believed to be useless!).

While it varies from person to person depending on several factors, in general the longer we're exposed to stress, the greater the risk of illness.

The National Institute for Occupational Safety and Health (NIOSH) estimates that 75 to 90 percent of office visits to a primary care physician are stress-related. Doctors used to believe that distress-related complaints were "all in your head," and to a degree they were right—because it does all begin in your brain. But the effects are very much in your body and can affect the way and the rate at which you age, and also predict not just the likelihood of catching a cold, but the diseases to which you may become susceptible.

Specific evidence of this was found three years ago when researchers at the University of California, San Francisco, uncovered signs of accelerated aging in mothers who cared for seriously ill children and felt they had little control over their lives.[20] Biological markers showed that these women were from nine to seventeen years "older" than their same-aged counterparts. The crux of the research lies in a part of a chromosome known as a telomere. As people advance through the aging process, the telomere begins to shrink and when it is too short to do its job effectively, the door to disease is left wide open. In this study, the longer women cared for the children the shorter their telomere became. Another aging variable was found in people who spent a hundred hours a week caring for a loved one with Alzheimer's disease.[21] In this instance, researchers found a dramatic increase in interleukin 6, a damaging substance in the blood that corresponded with levels seen in ninety-year-old people, even though the average age of the caregivers was only about seventy. In a similar group of caregivers, small wounds took nine days longer to heal than in non-caregivers.[22]

The undivided link between our brain and our organs is made crystal clear in cardiovascular (heart) disease, where the single best predictor of morbidity and mortality is not smoking history, diabetes, high blood pressure, or high cholesterol—but depression. The number of studies cementing the link between our emotions and our health could fill volumes. Take a look at just four of them:

- In a provocative project, reported in the *Journal of Occupational and Environmental Medicine,* researchers looked at the link between job stress, feelings of control, social support, inflammation, and infection in 892 male workers. More than all other risk factors such as smoking, cholesterol, or even blood pressure, it was stress and feelings of lack of control that predisposed the men to developing high levels of fibrinogen, a substance linked to an increase in blood clotting, heart disease, and stroke.[23]

- According to a study in *The Journal of the American Medical Association,* an abundance of "negative" emotions literally doubles the risk for ischemia, a condition characterized by an insufficient blood supply to the heart, compared to those who have more "positive" emotions.[24]

- In a study following over twenty thousand people for eight years, the risk of stroke was found to be more related to psychological distress than cigarette smoking, blood pressure, obesity, heart attack history, diabetes, family history of stroke, or cholesterol level, according to a study in the journal *Neurology.*[25]

- Serious aggravation on the job or in the workplace, in situations where one has little control, appears to increase the risk of developing colon and rectal cancers. Reported in the journal *Epidemiology,* researchers found over five times the prevalence of colorectal cancer in people who had a ten-year history of work related problems, after accounting for diet and other factors previously associated with these types of cancer.[26]

The chilling effects of chronic stress are also tied to infertility, rheumatoid arthritis, asthma, infectious disease, diabetes, DNA damage, and even memory related disorders. (High levels of stress hormones can shrink the hippocampus, a horseshoe shaped part of the brain responsible for memory.) Even the way we are treated as children has an effect.

According to epidemiological studies (the branch of medicine that deals with the rates and causes of disease) involving thousands of people, the impact of being mistreated in childhood is linked to an increase in inflammation and more than twice the risk for some serious diseases in adulthood. One nine-year investigation revealed that men who face chronic stress at work or home have a 30 percent higher chance of dying from all causes.[27] Chronic stress and negative life events—including divorce, job loss, death of a loved one, and even an unwanted relocation—have been repeatedly shown to have adverse health effects and have even been linked to the development and progression of some types of cancer.[28] Research across the globe echoes these findings. In Finland, scientists evaluated greater than ten thousand women over a fifteen-year period, exploring the relationship between stressful life events and the risk of breast cancer. The results? "Our data suggest that (stressful) life events increase breast cancer risk independently of body mass index, weight change, alcohol use, smoking, and physical activity..."[29] Similar findings sparked Ohio University's ongoing investigation, "Stress and Immunity Breast Cancer Project," spearheaded by Professor Barbara Anderson. Overall, women with advanced breast cancer who have abnormal levels of the stress hormone cortisol die significantly sooner than women with normal levels.[30] (More later about these studies and how to put the odds back on your side.)

While no one can definitively identify the precise mechanism that would account for these results, stress has been found to lower our levels of antioxidants, and cellular studies of stressed and depressed patients also show a reduced number of natural killer cells that are vital to the detection and elimination of tumors. Another possible correlation was uncovered in a 2008 Queen's University study in Canada demonstrating a relationship between severe stress and breast cancer. In this case, sustained exposure to a type of stress hormone (hydrocortisone) decreased the expression of a tumor-suppressing gene.[31] In other words, the tumor was allowed to develop because stress hormones blocked the gene that would normally come to the rescue. Similarly, investigators discovered another stress hormone (norepinephrine) that promoted biochemical signals stimulating certain tumors to grow and spread.[32] And in an in vitro study (one that takes place in a test tube), a common stress hormone (cortisol) reduced the tumor-fighting potential of a unique gene by three times—that's 300 percent!

This could be a make or break issue if you happen to need cancer surgery. New research out of Tel-Aviv reports that the key to preventing cancer from recurring may lie in reducing stress hormones prior to surgery. Dr. Ben-Eliyahu Shamgar says that there is a narrow window of opportunity of only about a week after the removal of a tumor for the immune system to kick in and kill any remaining cancer cells that may be circulating.[33] Stress hormones interfere with that process. Imagine, just when you need your immune system to be functioning at its finest, the shock and impact of the diagnosis can interfere with your ability to get the maximum benefit from surgery!

As if that isn't enough, stress can even compromise your body's ability to respond to treatment. Researchers pinpointed epinephrine, another stress hormone, as the culprit causing changes in prostate and breast cancer cells that make them resistant to treatment.[34] On the other hand, researchers found that people with "upbeat moods" have lower cortisol levels and lower levels of "two proteins that indicate widespread inflammation in the body."[35] These findings are just part of the reason we offer instruction on stress reduction and relaxation before and after cancer treatment or surgery.

This surge of research has had its share of unintended consequences— I've addressed the most relevant in Popular Pitfalls at the end of this chapter. They're important, so don't miss them! In the meantime, it's important to know that none of the clinicians are saying stress causes cancer, or any other disease for that matter. But the mechanisms are clear: stress can modulate how the immune system works and set the stage for problems, increasing our vulnerability to disease. As we learned earlier, genetic research demonstrates that stress, diet, toxins, and other factors together can expose or turn on a series of genes that are not in our best interest. While what we succumb to is personal and individual, unrelenting stress can be the common denominator in a host of medical problems. Since stress hormones have consequences and all of our organs can respond psychosomatically, chronic stress can nudge you in a direction that is detrimental to your health. So you can discern how you might be affected, the next chapter will give you a valuable key to measure your own stress response and take control of stress hormones, reducing them on demand. In the meantime let's take a look at one more mystery and then examine the evidence of how we know for sure that we can make a difference.

Hormones of the Heart

You may be familiar with Proverbs 17:22, "A merry heart doeth good like a medicine, and a broken spirit dries the bones" (*King James Bible*). But who would ever think that hormones produced by the heart could cure cancer? The improbable connection between heart hormones and cancer arose out of personal loss and tragedy. A doctor in Tampa, Florida, David Vesely, watched as his wife died of breast cancer in 2002. Becoming convinced that hormones controlled cell growth, he decided to place hormones produced from the heart into cultures of cancer cells. As the chief of endocrinology, diabetes, and metabolism at the Veterans Hospital in Tampa, and also professor of medicine, molecular pharmacology, and physiology at the University of South Florida, Dr. Vesely began using colon, ovarian, breast, prostate, and pancreatic cancer cells in cultures with heart hormones and found that the heart hormones killed up to 97 percent of all cancers within only twenty-four hours.[36]

The next phase involved mice and, at the end of a single month, the heart hormones had eliminated cancer in 80 percent of the mice injected with pancreatic cancer and in 66 percent of the mice injected with breast cancer. Even the cancers that were not completely eradicated were reduced to a fraction of their original size. And of those, none died of cancer; all died of old age. Trials involving people will be next. While accounts such as these bring up more questions than answers, without a doubt, there is more going on within us than a chemical soup of chain reactions. Rather, a deep resonant consciousness with a language of its own puts in high relief the interrelationship between all of our parts. We may not have cracked the code for the entire alphabet, but the data is rich and robust, and worth far more than a casual glance.

How We Know: What Came Before

Long before we had all this evidence, before we could define and explore the specific pathways of cell-to-cell communication, and before we could design sophisticated studies, keen observers of human behavior noticed that survival—sometimes against extraordinary odds—wasn't necessarily random. Viktor Frankl, heroic survivor of four concentration camps, including the most infamous, Auschwitz, observed firsthand the links between self-worth, free will, and the ability to survive. As hate's ravenous appetite consumed his practice, his home, and the lives of most of his family, Frankl, a psychiatrist, began his seminal work that would later make its way into the universities and laboratories of the world. In his book *Man's Search for Meaning*, he makes clear that we have the power to determine our reality. He writes, "When we are no longer able to change a situation—we are challenged to change ourselves."[37] Other astute observers of the relationship of suffering and the choices we make to the outcomes we face, took note of what Frankl had to say.

...if the head and body are to be well you must begin by curing the mind: that is the first thing ... for this is the great error of our day in the treatment of the human body, that physicians separate the soul from the body.

—PLATO, *CHRONICLES*, 15 C.E.

Clinical psychologist Dr. Lawrence LeShan was one of them. In 1952 LeShan began working with cancer patients who were considered terminal, many with a prognosis of just a few months to live. As he began investigating the life history, personality, and the emotional functioning of patients with cancer, he looked for patterns and used these clues to compare with the results of people who were cancer-free. Through an elegant scientific method, he discovered distinct differences between the two groups. He then used that information to help individuals focus on how best to use the diagnosis as a turning point, rather than an end point, in their lives. (Far from denying the prognosis, patients used it as a point of leverage, as an opportunity to heal the past in the present.) While I'm drastically oversimplifying his approach, it's important to know that LeShan's patients began to use their remaining time in distinct ways that reflected their unique hopes and dreams. And then, surprising even LeShan himself, an amazing thing happened: patients stopped dying. Approximately half of the patients classified terminal went into long-term remission; the last time I saw him at a conference, many of these folks were still living. Not surprisingly, LeShan was on our advisory board at Getting Well and his book *Cancer as a Turning Point*[38] is now a classic in the field. (Dr. Jeanne Achterberg, a pioneering scientist in medicine and psychology, calls LeShan a "national treasure." Check out his fascinating book, referenced in the Resource Guide.)

That psychological factors could impact the immune system to such a degree was staggering. The science behind LeShan's work wasn't formulated yet, but it was about to be. In the 1960s, Stanford University psychiatrist George Solomon, M.D., noticed that his patients with rheumatoid arthritis experienced flare-ups during stressful times. Solomon reasoned that the immune system was negatively affected by stress and he designed a series of studies with rats that confirmed the relationship. In the 1970s, psychologist Robert Ader built on those early studies by using rats bred to have lupus (an autoimmune disease that can wreak havoc on multiple body systems). Just as Pavlov's dogs were conditioned to salivate at the ringing of a bell, Ader's rats were conditioned to tone down their immune system and their symptoms improved. (Ader would later pen the classic text on a brand new field: psychoneuroimmunology.)

The data hinted at a clear feedback loop between stress and physical well-being, which opened the way for further investigation. Then in 1981 neurobiologist David Felten, M.D., Ph.D., and recipient of a Mac-Arthur Foundation "genius award," scrutinized tissue slides under the microscope and stumbled upon nerve fibers—in the spleen. He describes the excitement—initially believing it was a mistake—upon his full realization of the momentous implications. In this single instant, the standard for understanding our biological systems was rendered obsolete—the immune system and the nervous system, organs and blood vessels, the brain and body were indeed interrelated.

All of this led to a genuine revolution in thinking when a few medical practitioners responded, took note of the relationship between stress and disease, and connected the dots to anecdotal evidence in their own lives and in the lives of their patients. Prominent among these is Yale pediatric and general surgeon Bernie Siegel, founder of ECaP, whose best-selling books chronicle the collective effect of group support, attitude, self-acceptance, and improbable recoveries.

The energy was contagious. Likeminded groups began popping up and stories of remarkable recoveries spread. Soon claims were made, controversy ensued, and tempers flared—giving rise to a sophisticated analysis, which was initially conceived to prove that supportive therapy groups had no affect on longevity. Dr. David Spiegel of Stanford University reported in *The Lancet*, "We intended, in particular, to examine the often overstated claims made by those who teach cancer patients that the right mental attitude will help to conquer the disease."[39] What happened next was a pivotal moment that changed the face of cancer care. Using uncompromising scientific protocols, all eighty-six patients in this study faced a dire prognosis (stage III and stage IV breast cancer) and each received standard cancer treatment. As the study was "blinded," the treating physicians did not know which women were attending the support group and which were not. In the support group meetings, led by a health professional, the women were encouraged to honestly and freely discuss their feelings, including their distress, and support each other. They were also taught skills for relaxation. When the study concluded ten years later in 1989, researchers discovered that the women participating in the therapy group lived twice as long as those in the control group.

This was big news. John Hopkins, MD Anderson, and Memorial Sloan Kettering and other progressive treatment centers stepped up to the plate and began offering therapeutic support groups. Other studies ensued. Fawzy I. Fawzy, professor of the department of psychiatry and biobehavioral sciences at the David Geffen School of Medicine, UCLA, and associate director at UCLA's Neuropsychiatric Institute, specializes in the effect psychological factors have on cancer. In a trial with sixty-eight melanoma patients, Fawzy provided group support in a six-week program that included relaxation training along with techniques designed to replace faulty thinking. The participants, like the women in Spiegel's study, lived significantly longer and had half the rate of recurrence of the group who did not participate.[40]

Bearing this out is a series of rigorous investigations published over the past ten years demonstrating distinct physical benefits from such programs. At Ohio State University, hundreds of women receiving standard treatment for stage II or stage III breast cancer participated in groups that offered not only social support, but training in relaxation, stress reduction, coping strategies and encouragement to exercise.[41] Participants were found to have lower levels of stress hormones, improved immunity, and higher levels of an antibody that actively fights breast cancer cells than non-participants.[42] In an interview with *Science Daily*, lead investigator and Professor of Psychology Barbara Andersen said, "The bright and encouraging news is that psychological interventions have reliable biological effects that can benefit women with breast cancer."[43]

Extending the idea, similar research programs are tackling a variety of health issues. While reviewing this chapter, I came across a pilot study for people suffering from IBS (irritable bowel syndrome) using a home-based program with some of the features you'll find here.[44] Currently there are no reliable medications to treat all of the symptoms of this chronic condition. But in this study, supplemented by only four in-office sessions, 70 percent of patients reported significant improvement compared to only 7.5 percent of the non-participating group.

Not all results, though, are so conclusive, leading to sometimes vigorous debates. For a thorough critique of the more controversial studies, researcher and science writer Henry Dreher carefully examines the evidence in his recent work, *Mind-Body Unity*. His conclusion? While it is true that survival is determined by many variables, it is clear that coping style matters. Dreher explains: "If … [someone's] psychological handling of the stress of cancer had a 10 percent influence on his recovery, then it would be no small matter. 'In a tight election,' said [the philosopher Ken Wilber] 10 percent can make all the difference in the world.'"[45]

There's no need to wait for all the data to come in before we begin upgrading the quality of our lives. Dr. Goldklang, cancer specialist, adds, "Of all the things patients can do to help empower themselves, taking advantage of the mind-body connection appears to be the most important. Harnessing the energy of the mind promotes healing of the body and we want to do everything we can to achieve the best results." With that goal in mind, each successive chapter will deepen your understanding, expand your knowledge, and sharpen your skills. Sometimes a single factor is all it takes. Nicholas Hall, the PNI specialist you met earlier observes that it takes three things to get sick: 1. a biological event; 2. an environmental trigger; and 3. the genetic potential. Like the perfect storm, all factors have to occur at the same time. Altering one or more of those factors can make all the difference in the world in terms of health and longevity. The very next chapter will give us a tool to address that.

There is a Zen saying, "The unaimed arrow never hits its mark." Let's begin!

෪ව

POPULAR PITFALL #1: THE MYTH OF THE
POSITIVE ATTITUDE & THE DANGER OF PHONY PEP TALKS

Crying wasn't always the private matter it is today. Funeral rites in ancient Rome included collecting tears into small vials that were then buried with the deceased. The tradition made its way into the Victorian period where tears were collected in corked bottles. Jerry Springer and reality TV notwithstanding, our culture generally champions the notion "never let them see you sweat or cry." But according to Dr. Frey, a biochemist and director of the Psychiatry Research Laboratories at St. Paul–Ramsey Medical Center, our stiff upper lip may come at a high price. Studies he has conducted show that not all the tears we shed are created equal.[46] The tears we cry from physical discomfort (a stubbed toe, for example) and the tears we cry from emotional pain are chemically distinct from one another. The emotional tears appear to release toxins or waste products, possibly at least one reason most people feel better after a good cry.

Since feelings of sadness, anger, or irritability after a diagnosis are perfectly normal and even expected, how does this square with media reports touting the importance of a positive attitude? The confusion lies in the definition. For most, a positive attitude means adopting a cheerful, chin-up stance, often under the mistaken impression that negative thoughts or emotions, in and of themselves, are harmful to our health. In research and clinical settings, though, a "positive attitude" actually refers to embracing and experiencing the full range of human emotions, including the more challenging ones. This means neither denying nor indulging more difficult or "negative" emotional states but working through them, eventually transcending them, as we move toward becoming authentically hopeful, joyful, or confident. This rules out adopting a rigidly cheerful demeanor or an uncompromising Pollyanna attitude as a healthy coping strategy.

Untangling this common misconception is critical. Roger E. Dafter, Ph.D., the associate director of the Mind/Body Medicine Group at the UCLA School of Medicine, finds the idea that negative emotions are bad for the immune system and that positive emotions are beneficial for the immune system to be "simplistic, inadequate, and unsubstantiated."[47] He reports that research indicates emotions are actually necessary information, which ultimately helps the process of fighting disease and healing.

Erroneous information about the danger of negative emotions causes people to feel guilty for crying or feeling angry. Experiencing these feelings is not the problem; it is only when you habitually block feelings from your awareness that they impact your immune system in a less than optimal way. According to Pennsylvania State University psychologist Alicia A. Grandey, a variety of physical illnesses have been linked with suppressing emotions.[48] On the level of well-being, for example, suppressed anger eventually leads to resentment; unidentified fear progresses to panic; and chronic hopelessness deepens into depression. Researchers such as Jeanne Achterberg and Lydia Temoshok have demonstrated that suppressed anger and seeing oneself as a victim can also affect immunity. Supporting that picture, one recent investigation discovered a link between inhibited anger and an increase in pain severity.[49]

Armed with an accurate definition and a bit of practice, we can learn to interpret feelings as important messages. Though most of us prefer to be joyful and happy rather than annoyed or angry, these less than comfortable feelings motivate and inspire us to change the very conditions that created the discomfort in the first place. Paying attention to the message behind the feeling is liberating and very different from venting, raging, or hiding under the covers for weeks at a time. Appreciating the importance of experiencing all of one's feelings—and working through them—is empowering. Someone once said, "What you feel you can heal," and so it is.

彡ﾍ

POPULAR PITFALL #2: HOW STATISTICS CAN LIE

British Prime Minister Benjamin Disraeli is said to have written that there are three kinds of lies: "lies, damned lies, and statistics." And if this is true, nowhere does it have more impact than in the prognosis of serious illness. It's easy to become disheartened when facing a dire prognosis. Becoming educated on what statistics really mean for treatment and survival helps us embrace the idea that realistic doesn't mean pessimistic.

Since many beat the odds—either by surviving an "incurable" disease or by living far longer than expected—several cancer specialists refuse to give people the sentence of how long they have left to live. Rather, oncologists Gerry Goldklang, of Georgia Cancer Treatment and Hematology Center, and Jeremy Geffen, of The Geffen Cancer and Research Center, educate patients on what the statistics are all about. First, statistical outcomes regarding treatment options for most conditions are based on large numbers of people and do not accurately reflect how you, as an individual, will respond to a particular treatment. While these studies help you and your specialist select a therapy that will suit your situation, the statistics do not apply to your personal odds for a cure. For example, if a particular protocol in a clinical trial was successful in 30 percent of patients, many people interpret that to mean that they have a 30 percent chance of the treatment working. Not so. This number entails the total number of people receiving treatment and includes people who are over one hundred years old and who may have smoked cigarettes for eighty years. Of that entire group, thirty out of a hundred people responded to treatment. For the thirty who responded, their statistical outcome was 100 percent. Sounds a little different now, doesn't it?

ℰᴎ

POPULAR PITFALL #3: "FALSE" HOPE

Some take exception to resources like *Spontaneous Remission* in the mistaken belief that such cases support "false" hope. But the very notion of false hope is an oxymoron. As you have witnessed so far, many things influence the possibility of beating the odds, such as getting an accurate diagnosis, taking action, and responding in a positive way to your own particular risk factors. All of which depend on hope. It is the basis for self-care, which is inextricably linked to our survival. Without hope, you might not go to a doctor right away, get a second opinion, submit to chemotherapy, or have surgery. Whether it's taking your medicine, reading this book, or washing your hands, the motivation behind these actions has to be hope. It is the foundation for all positive change, be it keeping your resolution to lose weight or getting a mammogram.

Rather than diluting hope, we should be cultivating it. Numerous studies indicate that individuals who are apathetic toward healing, who lack social support, and who have a passive coping style have reduced immunity.[50] Taking it a step further, an attitude of hopeless fatalism has been linked to an increase in mortality in almost all diseases.[51]Lee Berk, Ph.D., a pioneering medical researcher, has shown that positive anticipation increases endorphin levels (a mood chemical produced in the brain), which enhances natural killer cell activity, among other things.[52] In an interview, Dr. Berk spoke about the "biology of hope." "I looked up the definition of anticipation and found it and the word expectation are synonyms for the word hope. I said, 'Well, here is another piece of the puzzle and more artillery for patients and patient care. Why aren't we providing the anticipation, the hope that would benefit patients?'"[53] If we're not getting that message from our health care team, we are called to generate it for ourselves. Although none of us know how long we will live, hope allows us to recognize the choices we have, and motivates us to take action in our own behalf.

૪ઙ

POPULAR PITFALL #4: BLAMING THE VICTIM

Because of the sheer volume of literature that links stress, perception, or our behavior to illness, we have created an unfortunate dichotomy with unintended and unnecessary consequences. Which brings me to the fourth misconception, and that is feeling responsible for the illness. Popular psychology articles, the misinterpretation of data, and gross oversimplification have left in their wake people who see illness as a sort of punishment for not living or thinking correctly. This is not only untrue, it is a hindrance that encumbers the already overwhelmed, wasting valuable reserves required for the necessary and productive work of rallying resources and the development of a support system. While excessive and prolonged stress has consequences, it's vital to distinguish these consequences from punishments.

Let me state this clearly: illness is never a punishment; it is a loss. People don't give themselves an illness. Babies don't give themselves developmental disorders, children don't give themselves leukemia, and adults don't give themselves lymphoma. Even polar bears are cropping up with genetic mutations from excessive toxicity in their environment and at times it seems our food and water supplies warrant a skull and crossbones label. All of this needs to be kept in balance. Science writer Henry Dreher states it best, "If I breathe in asbestos particles, have I somehow issued them an invitation?"

Further complications can arise if an individual does heal and solely credits their recovery to a particular type of emotional work. Imagine a person who becomes well after focusing intently on forgiving others. If the illness comes back, that person might say that he or she must not have done a good enough job of forgiving. But if someone chooses to do

work in the area of forgiveness because it offers a richer, more rewarding way of being, then the entire process is beneficial and not at all laden
with the expectation of a cure or accompanied by its evil twin, personal
liability. Motivation becomes not a clean CT scan, but the experience of
inner peace.

Nurse educator Janet Quinn, Ph.D., teaches that while we are not
responsible for the illness, we are called to be responsive to it. Certainly,
there are many valuable lessons from having a serious illness, and there
are few greater motivators for personal growth and change than a catastrophic diagnosis. But blaming ourselves for the illness is very different
than choosing to learn from it. We want to embrace the lessons the illness offers, but keep in mind that we did not need the illness to learn the
lesson. In this self-nurturing climate we can focus and rally our resources to respond to the challenge of the illness itself. In the six-week class,
we look at what we can do with it, where we can go, and what we can do
together. The real issue here is what we can do *now* to live better.

&ૠ 3 ૹ૭

Turning Stress into Strength:
Your Personal Key

Life is like a game of cards. The hand you are dealt is determinism; the way you play it is free will.

—JAWAHARLAL NEHRU
(FIRST PRIME MINISTER OF INDIA)

Just after midnight on Sunday August 31, 1997, a black Mercedes sped into the Pont de l'Alma tunnel in Paris. The driver, under the influence of a cocktail of alcohol and prescription drugs, nicked a white Fiat, spun out of control, and crashed into the thirteenth concrete support pillar inside the tunnel.

The details of events that conspired that night to take the life of Princess Diana are well known. But what if just one thing had been different? It could be the car, the state of the driver, the speed, a dark tunnel, paparazzi and cameras, booze and prescription drugs, or even the time of day. If just one of those risk factors were altered in this scenario, the outcome itself could be radically changed.

And so it is with us. In the last chapter you saw that while many factors influence our susceptibility to disease, it is the combined effects of genetics, stress, environmental toxins, infections, and injuries that create illness. Altering just one risk factor, though, can mean the difference between life and death. The biochemistry of stress fascinates scientists because unchecked stress hormones are major culprits in a host of disorders. Researchers say that stress-induced hormones flowing into the bloodstream in an uninterrupted course cripple the immune system, block processes that repair tissue, break down bone, and even act like battery acid on the memory center of the brain. It is as if we are stewing in our own juices. Yet before we can hope to stem the flow of stress hormones, let alone reverse it, we need to understand how stress changes us on the inside.

How Stress Can Save Your Life

Imagine that you are living in a part of the world where being chased by a tiger is a very real threat. As soon as you become aware of the tiger, a virtual pharmacy of biomolecular chemical reactions is activated. Your pupils open wider and even your peripheral vision is enhanced so you can take in every element of this danger—and maybe see the nearest tree to climb. As the tiger chases you, adrenaline courses through your body, elevating your heart rate and blood pressure, while arteries near your skin constrict so that more blood can flow to your heart. As your heart beats faster, blood is shunted from your hands and feet to your muscles, lungs, and brain so you can keep running faster and farther. If you are barefoot your feet might get cut and bleed, but your body knows that you can't afford to pay attention to such minor details right now, so feel-good chemicals (endorphins) hook up with opioid receptors (as in opium) to provide the perfect anesthesia.

To stay one step ahead of the tiger your body needs immediate energy, and digesting that super-sized burger and fries you just ate for lunch will only slow you down, diverting critical energy from the task at hand, which is to prevent *you* from being the super-sized lunch! Blood flow is shunted away from the digestive tract, as your body instinctively knows that now is not the time to use precious energy breaking down all those carbohydrates, proteins, and fats. Healthy digestion won't help you here. To gain its need for lightning fast access to glucose, your blood is flooded with insulin, which pushes the sugar into your brain and your hardworking muscles.

A full bladder could get in your way, so other hormones are released that curtail the production of urine by your kidneys. (In times of stress, other fluids are affected, too—if you ever wondered why you've had a dry mouth when doing something that makes you particularly nervous, like public speaking, now you know.) And fortunately, if you fall down and cut yourself or the tiger happens to bat you around a bit, an adrenal hormone called epinephrine comes to the rescue by making your platelets sticky—so you will be less likely to bleed to death. Later, having escaped with your life, your body will manufacture a smooth cocktail of sedatives to help you sleep. While sleeping, your breathing slows and deepens, and the reparative process heals you and restores balance to your brain and body.

How Stress Can Kill

The life-saving effects of the fight-or-flight response are both elegant and efficient—for short-term emergency use. But suppose the threat is not a tiger, or a speeding car, but merely the stress of daily life. In our society today, most of the stressors we experience are not occasional, sudden, or short, but are long, protracted, and continuous. The very same chemicals that helped us outrace the tiger, when persistent and prolonged, induce a macabre malfunction of our immune system. The thousands of possible diseases or conditions we may develop vary from person to person, depending on our unique threshold and genetics (some folks really are built to last!), but the fundamental cause remains the same: chronic inflammation from prolonged stress.

Inflammation, though, if you recall from high school biology, can be a good thing. In fact, if it weren't for the beneficial effects of inflammation, we would never heal a broken bone or stop a cut from bleeding. That cut, whether accidental or surgical, marshals a swift and sophisticated response. Specialized immune cells sniff out danger and rush to the scene, while others act like kamikaze pilots, engulfing bacteria and contaminants to keep you free from infection. And just to make the body's response to inflammation the best it can be, many white blood cells destroy unwanted invaders by secreting a type of bleach! Meanwhile, platelets clump together and seal off the bleeding while other cells create new collagen to repair the cut. In the visible world, you soon notice the obvious: a scab forms, the inflammation recedes, and you're good to go.

As a youngster, my stepson Matthew was a true protagonist against pain and suffering. If there was a way to avoid a situation where any possible pain or injury might occur, he'd find it. So when my husband went to get the tweezers to extract a splinter from my foot, Matthew pulled me aside and said, "Don't let him do it. I never tell anyone when I have a splinter because, if you just leave it alone, a callous will form and then it will gradually slough off and the splinter will go along with it." At first I just laughed but then I thought about the process of inflammation and by the time my husband returned with the tweezers I had decided to follow Matthew's advice. Sure enough, it got a little red and swollen. Inflammation was coming to my rescue, fending off disease-causing bacteria, and then the inflammatory process quietly receded. Just as Matthew predicted, a callous formed and before I knew it, there was no splinter.

Matthew was right about how the body normally heals, but what happens if the cells handling the injury don't stop? In that case, the result is chronic inflammation. Chronic inflammation is like a house of cards, destabilizing the natural repair process, instigating a self-defeating, vicious cycle that interacts with our genetic predisposition for disease. Fantastically complex, inflammation is the single underlying mechanism of the major killers of our time, scientists now believe— linking diseases as diverse as heart disease, osteoporosis, diabetes, Alzheimer's disease, and cancer.[54]

As you learned in chapter 1, this new view of stress and inflammation is changing the way we understand and treat almost every type of physical disorder and disease. Take, for example, the phenomenon known as Black Monday. More people suffer heart attacks on Monday morning between six a.m. and noon than at any other day or time of the week. Once a mystery, we now understand that sustained job stress, coupled with the melancholic business of the Monday morning return to the work week, can disrupt the cells that line your arteries, increase your blood pressure, and trigger blood clotting.[55] Previously, these changes protected you from the impact of an attacking tiger, but when they are chronic, they now put you at risk for a heart attack or stroke.

Even kidney damage and the bane of water retention can be caused by long-term stress. Stress hormones stimulate your adrenal glands to release steroids that cause sodium and water to be retained. Granted, a temporary decrease in urine output may be desirable, say while being chased by a tiger (no time for a potty break now!), but chronic retention of sodium and water cause swelling and can potentially damage your kidneys.

Diabetes and weight gain can often be directly linked to chronic stress. From your body's standpoint, when stress hormones are rampant, the goal is to stay one step ahead of the tiger, which, in real life, could just be a deadline or a cranky supervisor. In either case, your body believes that you are being "chased" or are under threat on a daily basis. To conserve energy, your metabolism is turned down and every available calorie is conserved. Digestive problems frequently develop (recall the reduced blood flow to your GI tract!) and chronically elevated insulin, which transported the glucose you needed when running from the tiger, now has the sinister effect of causing your body to store fat. This life-saving process, designed for short-term use, can in the long term lead to diabetes.

High levels of the stress hormone cortisol act like battery acid on the memory center of the brain.[56] Think about the last time you were rushing to get out the door only to discover that you had misplaced your car keys. Or perhaps your teenaged son has studied hard and is completely prepared for a chemistry final, but panics when taking the test and cannot recall what he already knows. Of course, these are only the short-term effects of cortisol. Excessive levels over a long period of time inhibit the creation of new brain cells[57] and can cause shrinkage of the hippocampus,[58] a part of your brain that plays an important role in memory and emotion, which is another reason why researchers link cortisol and excessive inflammation to Alzheimer's disease and other brain related disorders.

New Thinking on Illness

This radical perspective of what makes us sick has research and development centers of blockbuster pharmaceutical companies devoted to conquering this one problem: chronic inflammation. In each of these instances, unrelenting stress is the incendiary spark that fuels the fire of internal destruction.

New studies—synthesized from a number of scientific disciplines—are incredibly intriguing because they show us that under optimal circumstances immune cells swim through the bloodstream with speed and determination. Vigorous and unflagging, they are like little Pac-men devoted to their task of patrolling for and destroying bacteria and cancer cells before they multiply. But when the body is under stress, immune cells drastically slow down and their competence falters, allowing cancer cells to slip by undetected. More than cells are being studied, however. The scientific literature is packed with studies linking stress (likely mediated by certain biomarkers including cortisol and interleukins) to certain types of cancer.[59] For example, one provocative study found that women with a family history of breast cancer secrete more cortisol in response to daily stress than other women.[60] The process can be so silent that we may not even notice the steady crippling of our immune system until we are facing a dire diagnosis. When our bodies become so accustomed to high levels of stress and chronic inflammation, we may accept this lethal inner state to be normal. That is a dangerous illusion.

Consider this: If you were unkind enough to drop a live frog into a pot of boiling water, he would immediately try to jump out. But, if you put that same frog into a pan of cool water and gradually turned up the heat, he would stay where he was until he died. And so our poor frog has demonstrated the terrible effects of habituation—of becoming accustomed to something aversive to the point that we don't even notice it. Unfortunately, we humans may be more like this frog than we realize. Many newly diagnosed patients are surprised to discover that they, too, have unknowingly become habituated to the consequences of chronic, daily stress. Day after day they are manufacturing high levels of stress hormones even when they feel relatively free from external sources of stress.

The inconvenient truth is that most of us are plagued by a steady infusion of daily stress that is compounded by serious illness and more egregious burdens. When I first met Margaret at the cancer center, I discovered that her husband had walked out on her and their two children the week following her diagnosis of breast cancer. Between caring for her young children, recovering from surgery, and going back to work full-time, she had no time to replace the bar of soap she had been using in her bra to fill out the space her left breast had once occupied. Grappling with substantial obstacles, Margaret didn't need platitudes; she needed a quick and easy way to bolster her immune system while carrying on with the enormous task of living her life.

The Secret to Managing Stress

The good news is that you do not have to quit your job, retreat to an island paradise, or retire from life in order to reduce stress, because a single factor can change your biochemistry: the way you breathe. In spite of the fact that you take it for granted, your breathing is a kind of make-or-break process, a catalyst that either shifts you into a world of harmful hormones or into an impressive process of healing and repair. Shockingly effective, healthy breathing is the one thing that can reshape your biochemistry and bring you to higher levels of health and healing. Coming up, you'll learn a disarmingly simple breathing method that can be used anytime, anywhere, whenever you want to relax and recharge. But before reading further, notice how you are breathing right now.

Get Started Now: How You're Breathing

Put one hand on your chest and the other one on your abdomen. Notice which part of your body is moving by seeing if your chest or your abdomen rises and falls. Are you breathing through your chest (called thoracic breathing) or your abdomen (called diaphragmatic breathing)? If you struggle with cold or clammy hands, it has more to do with chest breathing than room temperature. (More about that coming up.) You may have a bit of movement in both areas. If so, see if you can focus on isolating your diaphragm, in which case only your abdomen will be moving and not your chest.

Unfortunately, you do not have to encounter an attacking tiger at all in order to find yourself in a "fight-or-flight" reaction. Just breathing high up in your chest is enough to trigger a cascade of stress hormones and a biological imperative that causes your body to react as if you really are facing danger, having insidious effects on your thinking. We automatically start scanning for problems, believing a serious threat might be lurking just around the corner. We can even invent problems if they aren't readily available! You can see how this works by imagining that all of your current cares and concerns have vanished with a magic eraser and your wildest dreams have come true. Perhaps you've won the sweepstakes and have retired to Tahiti, in fabulous health, of course. All of your loved ones are safe and in good spirits and you feel incredibly fulfilled. As you lie back in your hammock overlooking the coast, your breath begins to migrate from your abdomen up to your chest. As your breath becomes rapid and shallow, fight-or-flight hormones flood your body and suddenly you feel as if you've forgotten something important. Raising yourself up, you scan the horizon for sharks. Nothing there this time, but what about the shoreline? Doesn't that look like rapid erosion? What effect will it have on your beachfront property value? Maybe you should get busy and make a few calls to your realtor right away.

Put simply: regular chest breathing has serious negative consequences. Breathing this way, on a day-to-day basis, releases an arsenal of killer chemicals. Even when life is "perfect," if we are chest breathing, our bodies bear a burden that can negatively affect our health. Even our ability to enjoy the moment, or respond creatively to a challenge, is compromised since stress narrowly focuses our thinking and overwhelms our coping strategies.

How We Know: Controlling the Uncontrollable

Thankfully, you don't have to let this sort of stress short circuit you. As you may have already guessed, just as chest breathing causes a chemical cascade that has you looking for trouble, the reverse is true as well. Healthy breathing curtails the production of harmful hormones and generates healing ones, along with amazingly diverse, whole body health effects. For all of these reasons and more, elite athletes receive specific training in diaphragmatic, or abdominal, breathing. Plus, breathing in this way acts as a highly effective detoxification system, expelling the body's waste products on every exhalation. Internationally renowned cardiologist Stephen Sinatra urges patients to embrace healthy breathing:

> High-quality breathing is paramount to good health. If it is restricted, chaotic, or dysfunctional in any way, all other detoxification systems are impaired. The liver, colon, kidneys, and skin are commonly considered the major detox organs. To some extent, this is true, but the lungs are possibly more important to detoxification. When they are restricted, cellular activity is disturbed, and toxic buildup is increased. Over time, other organs of detoxification must fill in the gaps, which causes a greater burden to fall on them. …People who talk fast, interrupt others, suck in their breath, and generally don't pause, can create physiological damage to their bodies due to irregular breathing. A study conducted in Poland showed that these chaotic breathing habits cause the release of excessive amounts of a chemical that can predispose us to excessive inflammation.[61]

When toxins rise, the glands in your body can become overwhelmed and sluggish. Healthy breathing, though, can help dissipate toxic overload more quickly. J.W. Shields, M.D., writes that, "Deep diaphragmatic breathing stimulates the cleansing of the lymph system…[and] increases the rate of toxic elimination by as much as fifteen times the normal rate."[62] As you can see, beating the odds has a lot more to do with your lungs than you might have guessed. One reason for this is that our lungs have little air sacs called alveoli. If laid flat, end-to-end, they would cover a tennis court. When we are chest breathing, only half of our alveoli are being used; we're playing with only half a court, as it were. If we begin to breathe diaphragmatically, nearly all of the alveoli in our lungs are used, greatly enhancing the oxygen in our bloodstream, organs, brain, and even our digestive tract. (Children and adults who have asthma are taught this breathing method in order to expand their lung capacity and reduce the severity of asthma attacks.[63]) For those with cancer, the implications are profound: P.E.T. scans take advantage of the fact that many cancer cells derive energy by fermenting glucose in an oxygen poor environment.

When we are healing, the body's demands for extra energy and vital nutrients rise sharply. In order to efficiently convert food and fat into energy, the body's acid/alkaline balance needs to be maintained. Since oxygen is alkaline, deep breathing helps restore the optimal pH level for energy production. Enzymes, too, are sensitive to pH. The better our pH, the better our digestion and absorption of essential vitamins and minerals. (The lining of our digestive tract has little finger-like projections called intestinal villi; their job is to absorb nutrients, but to function optimally they need oxygen—and when we chest breathe they suffer.) Not to mention that chest breathing shuts down digestion, and when recovering from illness or surgery, we need more nutrients, not less!

This subtle practice has major effects. Studies show that people with type II diabetes are better able to regulate blood sugar levels—and lower death rate from all causes—with relaxation training, using some of the techniques coming up, including healthy breathing.[64] Other exciting reports indicate that regularly carving out time to meditate or mindfully breathe (focusing on your breath, not your problems) can help slow age-related memory deterioration and even brain shrinkage.[65]

Diaphragmatic breathing has also been successful in regulating heart rate in atrial fibrillation—where the heart beats rapidly and irregularly. One case reported by Dr. Andrew Weil[66] is that of a Chicago stock trader whose episodes of atrial fibrillation necessitated emergency treatment and drug management. But after learning about the power of healthy breathing, he began practicing regularly and hasn't experienced a recurrence since. At the primary care practice where I work, many patients with high blood pressure are able to lower it by focusing on diaphragmatic breathing alone. Terry Dvorak didn't want to go on blood pressure medication and tried a variety of other remedies to lower his blood pressure, which seemed stuck at 150/89. Terry wrote me that he had "tried herbs, blueberries, pomegranate juice, but nothing worked. Then my primary care doctor recommended a breathing technique where you breathe like a baby, using your stomach, and I thought I would try it. The results were dramatic. Now when I take my blood pressure, I sit down for a minute or so and breathe using my stomach muscles. My blood pressure has been 120/75, 124/78, and even 120/80. If I have trouble getting to sleep I use it and I go right to sleep." (There are even devices that feature interactive music and diaphragmatic breathing that can help lower blood pressure; see Resource Guide).[67]

There may be other life-saving benefits as well. A nineteen-year study at Yale University found that practicing meditation (featuring healthy, rhythmic breathing) just three times per week resulted in a 23 percent reduced death rate among older adults with high blood pressure, and decreased heart attack deaths by 30 percent and cancer deaths by 49 percent![68]

With a little practice, diaphragmatic breathing—not gulping air from your chest—is the one, simple, and everyday thing that you can do to turn daily activities into a wellspring of healing and inner strength. Like one woman said, "Wow! I love it—it's free, it has no negative side effects, I don't need Xanax to fall asleep anymore, and I can loosen my pants!" Broader benefits include enhanced sleep, extra energy, a greater sense of well-being, and the ability to navigate through the seemingly endless maze of tests or treatments with steady equilibrium. Healthy breathing is re-energizing and even massages your internal organs, improves blood pressure and resting heart rate, and reduces your risk of heart disease. The potential benefits are so impressive that health psychologists at Harvard Medical School are now beginning to go into the public school system to teach educators and students these methods.

Even more compelling is the control you can gain over your body by breathing in a healthy way. Once upon a time it was believed that functions of your autonomic nervous system (like heartbeat, blood pressure, and intestinal contractions) were beyond an individual's conscious control. We now know that this isn't true. Even rats can do it. In one experiment, rats were reinforced or trained to raise their blood pressure in one ear and lower it in the other. These little rodents had one bright red ear and the other pale and blanched![69] As you can see, people, much like these mice, can also be conditioned to control their autonomic reactions.

The first time I attempted something like this, I learned an important lesson in the process. Dr. Rita Stucky, a clinical psychologist, attached a temperature gauge to each of my hands. She instructed me to make the temperature of my hands rise by using only my mental powers. The harder I tried, the more the temperature dropped; my hands became colder by the second! And that's when I learned the secret of passive volition. Easily put, it's the opposite of trying too hard. In this case, using passive volition, my goal would be to create an intention (volition) and then release it or use a simple suggestion to gently bring it into play. To warm my hands with this principle in mind, I imagined a *warm* day at the beach, my hands resting on the *warm* sand.

A client of mine is a professional golfer. He explained to me that folks hone their skills on the driving range through repetition and practice. Then, when they go out on the golf course, they try too hard and lose control of the game. He said when on the course, the key is to let muscle memory and the subconscious take over. "It will take over," he insists, "if you let it." Trying too hard at anything makes it more difficult. It's true in the world of sports, the arts, and it's true in the world of healing. Trying too hard sabotages your efforts to heal by raising the very stress hormones you're trying to reduce. In the same vein, getting anxious about getting well interferes with recovery. On the other hand, using passive volition, you set your intention on your goal—say to heal or to warm your hands—but you hold it lightly in your thoughts, almost to the side. (You can see for yourself how this works by listening to the autogenic exercise on my website at www.brendastockdale.com.)

Gone with Girdles!

Relearning how to breathe may take some practice. Of course, when we were born we all started out breathing with our diaphragm. You can easily spot the little tummies of babies—or puppies—moving up and down. Somewhere along the way, particularly for women, many of us gradually began chest breathing and have to become reacquainted with abdominal breathing.

This isn't surprising considering our history of corsets and girdles. Watching the swooning spells of Vivien Leigh in *Gone with the Wind* or Keira Knightley in *Pirates of the Caribbean*, we are reminded that it wasn't so long ago that whale bone corsets were the order of the day. In the Victorian era, fainting couches were appropriately named, for if a woman wearing a corset exerted herself or received any sort of a shock, she simply could not take a full breath of air and would, of course, faint.

But clothing today isn't especially breathing-friendly either, and the culture reinforces it—if you can't hold it in, we have shaper panty hose and spandex girdles that can do it for you. Just holding in your stomach or wearing clothing that is too tight makes diaphragmatic breathing next to impossible, since holding in your stomach forces you to breathe with your chest. (By now, of course, you realize that holding in your stomach is really counterproductive because chest breathing will just increase any weight gain you're trying to hide.) Men I have worked with who consistently breathe with their chest often have military backgrounds (or a parent in the military) since the military posture demands holding in the stomach while sticking out the chest. This might make for a neatly regimented marching band, but it's not good for our health.

By simply observing your breathing style, you can learn a lot about yourself. Notice how you breathe when you are very relaxed or sleepy. It could be slow, deep, and regular. Then become aware of how your breathing changes when you are hurried, rushed, or angry—it might be rapid, shallow, and irregular. Harvard scientist, researcher, medical school instructor, and best-selling author Joan Borysenko teaches the importance of healthy breathing and recently took the time to share with me the way she uses the practice in her life. She said it works less well if she's in a grumpy mood (something hard to imagine listening to her melodious voice or seeing her radiant smile) but does the trick when she's feeling acute distress, whether cut off in traffic or reading an upsetting email. "I feel my body tense up and that's my cue to breathe properly."

Recently, while sitting in her car, "minding my own business...a crazed speed freak flew by on the right. Suddenly veering in front of me into the left lane, he inserted his giant black truck into a practically non-existent space between two cars. ...Surprise and anger flooded my unsuspecting body and mind as the whole left lane braked in unison to avoid a pile-up. I began to (chest) breathe like a freight train. It didn't help. ...I was tempted to forget my manners and chase the offender, but neither my rented Econocar nor driving skills were up to the task. Fortunately, I knew a less incendiary way to end the encounter. I did a minute of belly breathing and recovered my sanity. ...Breathing, after all, is the single most important skill for calming body and mind. ... Proper breathing is...the royal road to calming down and returning your body to balance."

It's no wonder that healthy breathing is taught in Harvard's eight-week mind-body medicine class. Joan explained that while some of the techniques are dropped when the class is over, all of the participants report using proper breathing frequently. "You don't have to make time for it, and you can do it wherever you are, getting the most of the proverbial bang for the buck. Nowhere is it inappropriate to breathe unless you're under water. It's the most natural of all natural functions and anyone can do it. Belly breathing isn't brain surgery. ...Make a few *Save Your Breath* signs on note cards and post them where you will see them. Make it a habit of checking on your breathing often, particularly when you feel rushed or overwhelmed. Let go with a sigh of relief, and then concentrate on five or ten belly breaths. Think of this as feeling the way to your 'sane center.' Over time, that feeling will become familiar, like home. You will find it easier and easier to experience peace."

Before belly breathing becomes second-nature you may find yourself yawning more than usual. But it's temporary! I know people are truly chronic chest breathers when they complain that they feel sleepy when practicing diaphragmatic breathing. When you are asleep, your breathing automatically shifts to your abdomen (unless, of course, you are having a bad dream). If the only time you are breathing this way is when you are sleeping, your body associates diaphragmatic breathing with being asleep. Until your body makes a new reference—that you can be alert *and* relaxed—you'll want to save your practice for when you're lounging at home. It's simply a matter of reconnecting to that breath and consciously implementing it on a daily basis. Soon you'll be aware and breathing, with energy to spare. In the meantime, start experimenting with your own healthy breathing.

Get Started Now: The Healing Breath

If you have primarily been a chest breather, when practicing this exercise, be sure to sit or lie down until your lungs and diaphragm are stronger. The sudden increase of oxygen in your brain can make you dizzy. Once you've become accustomed to it, the extra oxygen will carry you through the day without the early afternoon, foggy-headed feeling, or headache that comes from oxygen deprivation.

Get a medium-sized book and find a comfortable place to lie down.

Place the book on your abdomen and imagine for a moment that you are in a peaceful, relaxing place. As you do so, breathe in and out normally.

Notice if the book is wobbling or falling off to the side. If so, congratulations! You are breathing diaphragmatically. Scan the other points here and finish up with the Double Check at the end. If not, it is likely that you are breathing from your chest.

If you are a chest breather:

Again, do not try this standing up—make sure you are lying down! As you breathe in, pretend that your abdomen is like a balloon filling with air. As you breathe in, the balloon expands. Breathing out, the balloon deflates. (When I was first practicing, Dr. Stucky, who was teaching me, said I was just pushing out my stomach!) Be careful not to gulp air and stick your chest out. The goal is for your chest to be still with only your tummy rising and falling.

Speed things up by working with what is natural. Recall that your breathing naturally moves to your abdomen when you are sleeping. Take advantage of this fact and posture yourself for sleep. Put your feet up and watch a boring movie or read a slow moving book. As you begin to feel drowsy, pay close attention to your breath. Before you actually fall asleep, it will move to your abdomen.

Now you have a conscious awareness of what it feels like. Bring this awareness into your everyday life. Keep practicing. Breathe slowly and take breaks. With time it will feel completely natural.

If you are yawning:

Even if you are beginning to notice your abdomen rising and falling, if you feel the need to yawn it is a sign that you're not getting a complete exchange of oxygen and carbon dioxide. That's okay. Yawn, come up for air, and breathe like you usually do for a moment. Then try again.

If you are feeling sleepy:

This is a clue that you might be a chronic chest breather. If so, your body associates healthy breathing with sound sleep. Soon, though, your body will learn that you can be relaxed *and* alert!

Double Check:

Commonly, when I see patients the following week after learning about breathing, one or two people will believe they are breathing diaphragmatically when they are not. Make sure this isn't you! Sit in front of a mirror and put one hand on your chest and one on your abdomen. Be certain that the hand on your chest is still and that your abdomen rises and falls easily. Keep in mind that tears or coughing can be a release and a natural response to relaxation.

For a great website on healthy breathing see the Resource Guide.

Overcoming the Past

Most everyone who begins healthy breathing really enjoys the feeling of peaceful well-being. A few, though, experience almost a discomfort without being stimulated. Addicted to an alarm state that keeps them feeling super-charged, the feelings of relaxation that come from dia-phragmatic breathing are unfamiliar and not necessarily pleasant. They might feel restless or be consumed with distracting inner chatter.

Others don't feel safe with the sensation of being deeply at ease. Chil-dren who grow up in a spring-loaded environment where they are con-sistently criticized or abused have a constant need to remain vigilant and, since this sort of breathing releases feel-good hormones, it strikes an unfamiliar chord. Not surprisingly, they have higher rates of illness as adults than those who have not been subjected to this kind of early conditioning.[70] Repetitive damaging experiences seem to expose genetic weak points and exploit them, possibly by injuring the hypothalamus (a major control center of the brain) or inducing epigenetic change. Evi-dence, though, supports the idea that the damage can be overcome. Since our immune cells perform best in an environment that supports con-fidence and calm, and healthy breathing helps regulate the autonomic nervous system, gaining mastery over this important system can have dramatic and immediate benefits. One physician often writes instruc-tions for diaphragmatic breathing on a prescription pad. One woman calls it her "treatment." And so it is.

So don't give up! It took quite a bit of practice for me to be able to breathe abdominally and walk at the same time. I remember telling my doctor, "You have no idea how stressful it is learning to relax!" Over time, even for diehard chest breathers like me, the skill becomes auto-matic and reflexive. Even if you notice that you are frequently breath-ing from your chest, you will still experience the benefits if you take a moment to briefly refocus and begin breathing abdominally. A healing interval can even be as little as one minute every hour but even this small change produces big results. By interrupting the stress response throughout the day, your cortisol levels will be lower by the time you go to sleep, helping your body heal faster. Think about it: if your body spends all night trying to lower stress hormones, where does that leave your repair process? By keeping levels lower during the day, your body won't have to spend hours reducing cortisol to healthy levels but can immediately get on with the business of repair. In this way your sleep can be truly restorative.

As you've gathered by now, a tantalizing clue to your breathing pattern is how warm or cold your hands are. You may recall how the fight-or-flight process constricts blood flow in your extremities. Chest breathing is the major reason people have cold hands. Likewise, diaphragmatic breathing expands your capillaries and warms your hands. So, unless it's really freezing, your hand temperature says more about how you're breathing than the temperature of the room.

Controlling your hand temperature is easier than you think. Similar to mood rings from the seventies, inexpensive Biodots are tiny round dots that adhere to your hand. These quick acting, stress-measuring devices indicate temperature (blood flow) by turning color from black to blue or violet, and function as a very simple biofeedback device. A card defines the color range so you can see just how stressed out you are—or how well you are breathing. (See the Resource Guide to order.) Realizing that you can control blood flow in your fingers restores a sense of self-mastery and personal power, replacing the central insult of the helplessness that can sometimes accompany an illness. What brought all of this home to me more than anything, however, are the experiences of folks in my six-week classes. Our group members not only feel empowered, but also report diminished pain, better sleep, reduced anxiety, and fewer digestive problems. As they witness the overwhelmingly positive benefits in their lives, just from breathing, healthy new and solid connections to vitality and wellness are made. Stressed individuals with lowered immune functions are able to significantly alter their situation through verbal relaxation exercises and healthy breathing. Such radical transformation is possible for you, too.

A caveat: While cold hands are a true touchstone to indicate chest breathing, warm hands do not always signify the reverse. Some folks have nice, hot hands no matter how they're breathing; in which case, you'll have to rely on noticing whether your chest or abdomen is moving. And by the way, clammy, sweaty palms are also indicative of chest breathing. (Certain lie detector tests are based on this fact and measure subtle changes in the sympathetic nervous system that affect moisture.)

Breathing for Your Health

Everything becomes easier once your biochemistry is on your side. In an anxiety-provoking situation slow, rhythmic diaphragmatic breathing can help you think more clearly and stop the flow of panic-inducing chemicals in their tracks. (If you have panic attacks, breathing this way can be a quick fix.) And while facing a challenge, diaphragmatic breathing will expand your options and enhance your ability to deal creatively with whatever problem you are facing.

Diaphragmatic breathing allows for a reconstructive experience that actually builds new neuronal pathways and makes room for fresh interpretations. Once we're no longer stewing in our own juices we have more opportunity to respond differently to external demands. The self-soothing capacity of our breath allows us to choose how we *respond* to our circumstances rather than how we *react*. Just as in playing the hand that is dealt us, we determine whether we have a horrible experience or cope and transcend it. Even if the situation you are facing isn't likely to change or improve, diaphragmatic breathing will help keep harmful chemicals from wreaking havoc with your health while you are dealing with difficult circumstances.

You especially need the gift of your own breath when you are healing or facing weighty choices that have life and death consequences. At such times you simply cannot afford for your brain to be flooded with fight-or-flight chemicals that block your inner awareness and guidance system. Being in touch with your gut instinct has special advantages. Your intestines and digestive system have more nerve cells than your spinal column, which is one reason why the gut is called the second brain. Shallow breathing interferes with this intuitive and valuable source of information, while deep breathing, with its healing power can illuminate the choices you have and refine how you make them. At the very least, your ability to feel appreciation or gratitude is blocked if you believe a tiger is chasing you.

Stop Losing Energy Now!

Another desirable side effect of diaphragmatic breathing is that it helps you relax your muscles and conserve your energy. Chest breathing for extended periods can cause an excessive loss of carbon dioxide (CO_2) that causes the pH of the blood to rise too high (called respiratory alkalosis). This causes a biomechanical stress on the neck and shoulders as they work harder to support thoracic breathing.

Imagine, for example, two administrative assistants. Both are under time pressure to quickly produce a large amount of typing. One is sitting close to the edge of her chair, legs flexed, shoulders raised slightly. As she focuses on the material, her eyebrows knit together, and her jaw is clenched. She feels rushed and harried. The other is relaxed in her chair, back supported, shoulders relaxed, legs relaxed or gently crossed at the ankles. Her jaw is loose and a slight smile relaxes her face. She is working steadily but in no particular hurry. Who do you think will make fewer mistakes? At the end of the day, who will be more likely to enjoy her evening? It is easy to see that the first assistant consumed a tremendous amount of energy in simple nervous tension. That energy won't be available to her after work to exercise, play, or concentrate on a hobby. Understandably, she'll probably have to spend her evening recovering from a headache. On the other hand, the second assistant used only the energy necessary, primarily in her arms and fingers, to complete the job. She'll have a reservoir of energy that she can use for any number of things: healing, restoring balance, or playing a game of tennis.

There's a lesson for all of us in this example: rather than wasting energy in useless muscle tension,[71] practice using only the degree of energy a task requires along with your healthy breathing. In waiting rooms of doctors' offices, during CT scans and MRIs, and other common situations where waiting is customary, use each opportunity to close your eyes, breathe, and relax. You have the power to turn even stressful and potentially agitating moments into a healing experience.

Relax—On Cue

Once you have developed and strengthened this skill, as an added bonus, you can take advantage of a cueing technique to help you instantly relax. Just as Pavlov taught his dogs to salivate to a bell, it is possible to teach your autonomic nervous system—even your immune system—to respond in a certain way. Your posture or movements and your breathing are entwined in a beautiful equation, and in a sense, tell your brain how you should feel. Given your unique history, your brain comes to associate particular movements (and breathing patterns) with certain physiological states.

A friend of mine, for example, taps her foot or jiggles her leg whenever she feels uptight. She's been doing it for so long that all she has to do is start tapping and she's on a fast track to tension and stress. In the same way, you can make this kind of trigger work for you by training yourself to use a particular motion to bring about a feeling of well-being. Every time you are peaceful and deeply relaxed, simply place your hand over your heart or bring your thumb and forefinger together. In time your body will respond to the cues on demand, so if you are facing a deadline or find yourself in a business meeting where tension is high, you can touch your fingers together and your body will begin to relax. The touch becomes your cue.

Of course, any simple, reproducible movement or posture will work—even putting your finger on the tip of your nose—but most people prefer something a bit less obtrusive. Some people prefer using a small vial of a particular scent or essential oil that they enjoy. Smelling this scent while relaxing can, over time, induce the relaxation response by just breathing in the aroma. In short, anything can serve as a cue if you associate it with relaxation and feelings of well-being.

Just as you can make a big difference by small changes in your breathing, another factor that leads to health and healing is what you feed your mind or how you think. Whether your stress is real or imagined is irrelevant. It has the same effect on your body. Remember our illustration about being chased by a tiger? What if after running some distance you turned around and discovered it was not a tiger after all, but a kitten? Although all along it had just been a kitten, your physiological response was based entirely upon your beliefs and your perceptions! It goes both ways. Just as chest breathing triggers a flood of damaging hormones, thinking about or believing that a threat exists is enough to initiate the complete stress reaction. It could even be as innocent as lounging in your hammock by the Pacific Ocean while thinking about all the work piling up on your desk in Ohio. You'll get the best result when you do both: practice healthy breathing and choose your thoughts wisely. Later you'll be introduced to some tricks of the trade that help harmonize your thinking, but in the meantime our thinking can create images or pictures in our minds that have physical consequences. This is why we can imagine, for example, losing someone close to us, and tears will begin to form. This is the secret of Hollywood's success. The big screen transports us to a world where something we know is not real, yet causes us to catch our breath and alter our perception of reality. Your own imagination acts in exactly the same way. You will discover just how powerful your imagination really is and how it can help you heal in the next chapter.

Week Two

❧ 4 ❧

The Healing Power of Imagination: Technology at Its Best!

We must learn imagery is everything. We create our world or it is created for us. We will be effects if we are not effectors, victims instead of masters of our destiny.

—PATRICIA NORRIS, PH.D.,
OF THE MENNINGER CLINIC

Gary was eleven years old when an aggressive brain tumor first threatened his life. Despite two surgeries, by the time he was thirteen it had become inoperable. As the tumor continued to grow, Gary eventually lost the vision in his right eye, then the use of one leg, and finally the other. Partially paralyzed and unable to attend school any longer, he used a skateboard to scoot around the house on his elbows. But Gary's father refused to relinquish hope. He continued to research options and possibilities that might save the life of his young son. And by the time the doctors told him that Gary wouldn't live past Christmas, he had stumbled upon the Getting Well program in Orlando, Florida.

Gary was intrepid. Even though participating would land him in a group made up entirely of older women, he was willing to give it a try. He shared fully in the stress management exercises, contributed his own thoughts and ideas to discussions on finding meaning in suffering, and didn't try to get out of art therapy. So when it came time to learn a relaxation technique featuring his imagination, there was no holding back.

Imagining his white blood cells as powerful spaceships and his tumor as a stupid, evil planet that needed to be destroyed, Gary slowly began to improve. Christmas came and went, and he began to regain the use of his legs. Tests showed the tumor was shrinking. Soon, he went back to school. About a year later, his doctor told him that the tumor was as flat as a pancake and ready to be absorbed by his body. When Gary turned sixteen, local TV networks in Mobile, Alabama, filmed him getting his driver's license. At eighteen he played on a soccer team in high school and when he was in college his story captured the attention of national media. Shying from the limelight and grateful for every moment, Gary later found his calling near Billings, Montana, working on a ranch.

Enlisting the aid of your imagination isn't as farfetched as it might sound. The biological impact can even be measured. For example, just imagining lifting weights while your body is completely still and relaxed can actually increase muscle strength.[72] Additionally, pictures of the brain using positron emission tomography (PET) and functional magnetic resonance imaging (fMRI) reveal that visual images activate various areas of the brain in the same way the actual event would.[73] From there the vivid effects of imagination are distributed body-wide, the endocrine, immune, and autonomic nervous (which controls your breathing, heart rate, and blood pressure) systems are all affected.[74]

Gary's use of imagery is not a mysterious process. It's a technology we were born with that's partnered with us through every step and facet of our lives. Whether or not we've been aware of it, we access this technology on a daily basis, such as when deciding what to have for lunch, what to wear to work, or how to swing a golf club. Whether you see your choices in your mind's eye or feel your way through your options, imagery is involved. In fact, every time you access a memory you're using this technology in your own unique way. When you're deciding where to travel on vacation, you might reflect on your choices visually, get a sense of the type of trip you'd like to take, hear the music, or feel the waves, but in any case, I'll use the word *imagery* to describe all of that—whatever way you happen to use your imagination.

To see how you already use this natural process, think about a trip or a vacation that you took at some point in time. You may want to close your eyes to pinpoint a particular memory or it may be right there waiting for you. Got it? However you did it, that's imagery. Using imagery for health and recovery is just an extension of what you've already been doing, but now with awareness you can harness its power for your greater good.

How We Know: Your Imagination at Work

The reason this is so powerful is that as you imagine yourself in any given scenario, your body responds as if you were really there. The part of your brain that's engaged in this process doesn't distinguish between what you imagine and what is really happening. If you considered biting into a sour, juicy lemon as discussed in chapter 2, you might have salivated. Now you can take this further and get a sense of the power these images hold. Think about the last time you saw a scary or suspenseful movie at the theater. Let's use *Jaws* as an example. Do you remember the specific musical score just before the shark quietly ripped someone from below the surface or exploded out of the water? With the element of sonic suspense you might feel apprehensive and start holding your breath. Suddenly, something jumps out of the water—and you jump as well—maybe with a sharp intake of breath and a wild look of surprise in your eyes. It could just be the frog, like in the beginning of the movie, or later, the great shark himself. You might feel jittery or your hands could get clammy, but either way your conscious mind knows you willingly showed up for this, paying perhaps nine or ten dollars for the experience, plus you're sitting with dozens of other people and maybe even eating popcorn. The film isn't even in 3-D—and yet you jumped. You're not alone. It's the way we're designed and Hollywood counts on our response, called the willful suspension of disbelief.

It's one reason we can buy into and feel what is pictured on the big screen even though we know it's just a movie or why we can cry at the thought of a sad event, even though it may never happen, or feel excited imagining an upcoming adventure. When you use your imagination, your body experiences physiological changes as if the events were actually taking place in that very moment. We can exploit this natural process and consciously create a new chemical reality, one more suited to our purpose of healing.

In women who practiced imagery, researchers recently found significant differences in natural killer cell function—an important measure of immunity—compared with those who did not. In this case, investigators at the University of South Florida randomly assigned twenty-eight breast cancer patients to either a control group or an imagery and relaxation group. Both groups received traditional treatment, but four weeks later only the imagery group had heightened immune function.[75]

More research shows that imagery even has the power to affect the physical structure of the brain. In a compelling study at Harvard Medical School, volunteers learned a simple piano exercise. After practicing daily for five consecutive days, they took a test (transcranial-magnetic-stimulation or TMS) that allowed researchers to see how the motor cortex was affected—and sure enough—the more they practiced the piano exercise the more space the brain devoted to that area. Taking it a step further, another group of volunteers only imagined playing the piano piece, visualizing the finger movements but in reality, keeping their hands perfectly still. At the conclusion of the study, the motor cortex of the brain was expanded in exactly the same way as those who had actually played the piece![76]

The author of *What We May Be*, Piero Ferrucci, writes, "A six-year old girl ... having received a bicycle for Christmas started to ride it immediately, without any difficulty, before the astonished eyes of her parents. When they asked how she had learned to do that, she answered: "I had been imagining it all the time."[77] For decades, athletes have used imagery to enhance physical performance, practicing the sport in their mind's eye. Investigating the results of different practice methods, one group of basketball players practiced several days a week. A second group sat out but visualized themselves playing the game. The third group did nothing. At the end of the study, all three groups were evaluated on their skill level. Not surprisingly, the third group's performance was the lowest. But the performance of the imagery group was virtually indistinguishable from those that practiced several days a week.[78]

What I appreciate about imagery is that it's so efficient. According to the January 2008 Mayo Clinic Health Letter, the healing message is passed along to all the body systems, having a broad range of effects.[79] Visual images stimulate the optic cortex, imagining sounds influences the auditory cortex, and thinking about tactile sensations activates the sensory cortex. All of these interact with the limbic system, the emotional center of the brain that interconnects sensory networks with your endocrine, autonomic, nervous, and immune systems. This interconnectedness allows imagery to be your fast pass to all the perks.[80] Using all your senses, making your imagery richly evocative with a felt sense gives it more power.

At Vrije University in Amsterdam, psychologist Frank Bakker and colleagues hooked up thirty-nine men and women to machines that monitored electrical impulses in both arms. They first did six lateral arm raises holding either ten- or twenty-pound weights and then were told to remain still and imagine themselves doing the same lifts in two different ways. One was to watch themselves performing the exercises as if from a distance, and the second was to imagine the physical sensations that would normally accompany each repetition. Significantly more electrical activity was detected when subjects imagined the physical sensation of weightlifting. When using your imagination, create a luxurious experience by smelling the pine trees, feeling the smooth, cold rock, tasting the salt air, seeing the mist on the water, or listening to the waves as they crash upon the shore.

Taking advantage of this natural effect can give you a valuable edge when beating the odds. An extensive and compelling body of evidence demonstrates that imagery, with its power to evoke significant physical responses, can affect a wide range of health issues: heart rate, blood pressure, muscle tension, the allergy response, type II diabetes, asthma, coronary artery disease, headaches, hypertension, and irritable bowel syndrome. Imagery can reduce chemo induced nausea and vomiting, improve sleep and mood, relieve pain, and reset the body's thermostat (hypothalamic and autonomic regulation).[81] Recent research indicates that specific imagery targeting white blood cells—a key component of the immune system—has a direct effect on their function.[82] (It has even been used successfully in smoking cessation.[83]) An Australian review of the data showed that those using imagery or similar techniques had nearly 90 percent less heart disease, more than 50 percent less tumors and hospitalizations, and 30 percent less infectious diseases than those not using such methods.[84]

A recent report published in *Clinical Cardiology* made headlines when researchers from Yale University School of Medicine found that meditating three times per week for six weeks improved endothelial (cells throughout the circulatory system) function, and reduced blood pressure, resting heart rate, and the risk of heart disease.[85] In a similar study, scientists at the University of Iowa followed adults with high blood pressure for nineteen years. Those who meditated had a 30 percent decrease in heart attack deaths, and cancer deaths were reduced by 49 percent.[86] (See endnotes for additional studies.)

Martin Rossman, a physician who has taught imagery to thousands of patients and is the cofounder of the Academy for Guided Imagery, sums it up like this:

> I've seen many people with chronic illnesses find pain relief, better
> sleep, relief from anxiety and learn to live with much improved

health. I've seen heart disease being reversed and diabetes and hypertension go into remission with natural treatments. Most of my cancer patients go through treatments with much less discomfort, anxiety, nausea and fatigue than they did when there was no way to get them involved. I've seen many people survive diseases that they were told would kill them. On top of that, I've seen hundreds, maybe thousands of people who felt they were helpless victims of illness realize that they can play an active part in their healing, and find a great source of strength and pride when they do. They become aware that they are powerful, even if they are not omnipotent, and it makes a difference in their whole life, not just with their physical health. ...[87]

Gateway to Healing

Spotlighting other effects, some cancer centers and hospitals are introducing patients to imagery prior to surgery. In a 2007 study of Blue Cross/ Blue Shield members, those who used a guided imagery audiotape before surgery documented a substantial reduction in anxiety, were released from the hospital sooner, and had less postoperative pain and fewer complications.[88] (With what you learned in chapter 2 about reducing risks in cancer surgery, you can appreciate the further significance of the outcome.)

This is big news for insurance companies. An initial outlay of about forty dollars resulted in total cost savings of two thousand dollars per patient. "This finding," Dr. Rossman writes, "... has already stimulated the use of similar programs by other major health plans and medical groups. If similar results were achieved with a medication, it would be prescribed routinely by anesthesiologists and surgeons as part of a presurgical regimen, and I hope that this study will help us move toward the day when presurgical preparation using guided imagery becomes the standard of care."[89]

But you don't have to wait for your insurance company to get the message. In one of our programs a patient shared her own dramatic story about using imagery before surgery. Grace had inflammatory breast cancer, an aggressive type that infiltrates the lymphatic system. Chemotherapy had controlled but not cured the condition and a radical double mastectomy was the next step. Picturing her immune system as an Etch-a-Sketch she imagined the little wand gathering up all the magnetic shards (cancer cells) and directing them toward the nipple of each breast—only the nipple (she figured that since her breasts were to be surgically removed the nipples were the furthest point away from her body.) For a few weeks before the procedure Grace practiced her imagery at home with a particular piece of music and the added dimension of aromatherapy. Her surgeon agreed that Grace could bring both the music and the aromatherapy into the operating room. (Maintaining a good relationship with your medical team can go a long way.) A few days later, the surgeon called Grace, stunned and confounded by the tissue analysis—cancer was found nowhere except in the nipple of each breast!

Not every situation allows us to prepare ahead of time, though. Right after this particular session of the program (week two), Judy went to the hospital for an endometrial biopsy, which can be quite painful. She had just been introduced to these concepts and so she asked the doctor to pause for a moment while she did some diaphragmatic breathing and visited her "healing place" while intending that the entire area would be numb. She felt no pain during the procedure—her doctor was amazed and wanted to know how she did it. (For many, imagery offers another dimension to the practice of relaxation by creating a safe place and providing distance from pain.[90]) The following week she told us that since she had only learned about imagery that very day, she hadn't developed an image, but was able to change her physiology through breathing and setting an intention of being pain free.

At times imagery can serve as a bridge to treatment. A cancer specialist referred his patient Karen, who was unable to receive any more chemotherapy until her white cell count improved. As a nurse Karen was very much aware of her precarious situation, but she was also open-minded and willing to learn. After she was taught the basic steps and had practiced for a few days, an image popped into her mind of a Lawrence Welk bubble machine manufacturing an abundance of bubbles, symbolizing her white blood cells. Then she added the target number she was trying to reach. Karen began using this particular imagery on a Thursday. By Monday, her count was normal and she was able to receive chemotherapy.

As you can see, imagery is not a replacement for medical treatment but augments the care you are receiving. Along with your breathing it's a quick fix for changing the channel on hurry and worry so you can redirect that energy into healing. But you don't have to have a medical condition to benefit.[91] My father, as you read, is a scientist, grounded in the world of mathematics and equations and not inclined to poetic flights of fancy, yet he's a true believer in the power of imagination. At seventy-two he's hale and hearty—and every night before falling asleep he imagines his telomeres (a barometer of aging that shrinks as we get older) getting longer and he sees a graphic of a clock, with the hands turning backward in time until he reaches the age of thirty. (At first the hands of time went back to when he was a ten-year-old boy, but we teased him about not being able to keep secrets and said maybe that was why—after that, he stopped the hands at thirty!) A good friend of mine, Joy Hooper, tells me she practices these techniques so she "won't need a remarkable recovery!"

Personalizing Imagery

In these real life examples everyone's images are different and for a good reason. In the early days of photography, daguerreotypes were images captured on a silver-coated plate. Because there was no negative, all the photographs were originals. Like those early daguerreotypes, healing images are absolutely unique. You can see for yourself how this works in the following easy exercise. This isn't one to save for later—and since it only takes a minute—go ahead and try it now. You may want to read through it first, or simply take in a couple of sentences at a time, reflecting on them as you move through the exercise. Or if you like, you can listen to it on my website at www.brendastockdale.com.

Get Started Now: Your Healing Place

Spend a moment becoming quiet or just noticing your breath. When you're ready, in your mind's eye, allow yourself to visit a comfortable and refreshing place. It could be somewhere in nature, a physical residence, a favorite vacation spot, or a place that exists only in your imagination. If it seems good to you, take your time here and spend a moment exploring your surroundings. Notice the time of day. Is it early morning, afternoon, or dusk? Observe the sky and how the air feels against your skin. What time of year does it happen to be? Is it the crisp feeling of fall or the warm, humid air of summer that greets you here? Gently notice how your clothing feels against your body, the weight and texture of your garments. Allow the fragrance or aromas of this safe place to come into your awareness. It could be the fresh scent of pine or the salty smell of the ocean. There may even be a taste to the air. Notice the textures all around you. Perhaps you can touch the smooth, cool surface of a hard rock or feel the warm granular sand beneath your feet. Take in the image with all your senses. You may or may not see these things with your mind's eye, but you can sense them and you can know that they are there. Listen to the sounds of this special place. It might be ocean waves lapping the shore, the call of gulls, or the sound of pine needles crackling beneath your feet. Embrace this space with all of your senses and relax in the peace and safety offered here. Enjoy all the sights, sensations, and sounds of your healing corner of the world. And then when you are ready, slowly and gently bring your attention back to the room where you are and to the pages of this book.

If you try this exercise with ten different people, you will find ten different scenarios. Some love the beach; others enjoy the forest. For some, it is early morning in spring, while others are seeing themselves enjoying a snowcapped mountain peak in winter. The meaning we ascribe to places is as individual as we are, and, for this reason, imagery is a deeply personal process. Bringing this point home is a training program on the medical use of imagery at Harvard Medical School, where slides of cottages by a popular painter are flashed on a screen. Some in the audience find the paintings cozy and comfortable, yet others get a distinct

> *Imagination is more important than knowledge.*
>
> —ALBERT EINSTEIN

Hansel and Gretel feel about the very same pictures. In the same way, your images will differ from others even if facing similar problems. Gary, Grace, and Karen all had cancer but the context, the intent, and the image were all very different.

While guided imagery (where someone gives you an image) can be enormously helpful, the customizing element can be lost. For that reason, I've not given you a formula for various symptoms and disorders but rather a few simple steps and examples that will help jumpstart the process. Since imagery is extremely practical and can be used almost anywhere, designing your own imagery helps you internalize the process so you can take it with you wherever you go. As a tool or a skill it can help you adapt to any situation or problem you may face. You don't have to rely on a CD (circumstances may not allow it) or a facilitator (there may not be one when you need it most). And, as in Gary's case, personalizing your imagery offers a blueprint of what you want to achieve immunologically. The five steps below are based on radiation oncologist Carl Simonton and Stephanie Matthew-Simonton's approach for cancer patients[92] along with Drs. Jeanne Achterberg and Frank Lawlis, whose revolutionary work with imagery has been adapted to many different health challenges.[93] The steps here are followed by an example that brings it all together. Here are the five steps:

1. *First, we ask for an image or a metaphor of the problem or condition.* Doing this may require understanding your medical situation at

least in a cursory way. Take the complex condition of autoimmunity. A super simple picture or metaphor might be that the immune system has overreacted, attacking healthy tissue rather than just viruses and bacteria. One woman with multiple sclerosis saw little men with pick axes, symbolizing her "hyperactive and confused" immune system, tearing apart the drywall—her image for the myelin sheath. Then she saw the captain of the team (her brain!) redirecting the men to repair the entire area. Using drywall mud and plaster they created a beautiful finish. If a virus, bacteria, or cancer is the focus, you may want a symbol of your immune cells gobbling up little bits of trash or destroying it (like Gary's spaceships). For certain medical conditions looking at pictures of the organs involved may give you some helpful ideas. Having a playful attitude toward imagery keeps it relevant and relaxing, and counters any of the stress hormones associated with trying too hard, which you learned about in the previous chapter.

2. *And then we imagine the resolution or healing of the problem*, like the bubble machine or the Etch-a-Sketch. Likely the resolution will consist of your own immune system working optimally and efficiently, returning to a healthy balanced state. Sometimes steps one and two are entwined, as in the example of high blood pressure found in the book *Imagery for Getting Well*.[94] Here the author suggests a possible image of the blood—or scrubbing bubbles—moving through the body, expanding vessels, softening the walls, reducing clots, and eroding plaque. (For more ideas and intriguing characteristics of immune cells see "White Blood Cells: The Backbone of Your Immune System" on page 98.)

Keep in mind that since you're forming a blueprint of healing, you want to see the problem as completely resolved. At times patients in the program report seeing it "mostly healed," but this isn't the final goal they are really seeking. If you were designing a home to be custom built and the architect showed you the blueprint but there was no roof or the closets were missing would you say, "well, okay, we'll go with that, it's mostly done"? Hardly! The blueprint of what we want to occur is the complete resolution of the problem and the restoration of the body back into harmony and balance.

In the case of cancer, it's helpful to remember that our immune system has met that challenge before. Cancer cells pop up frequently in our bodies and under optimal conditions our immune system takes care of them. One oncologist reports that in the laboratory our own white blood cells are more powerful than cancer cells.[95]

So, having cancer cells is not the central problem; their unchecked growth and proliferation is. In autoimmunity the good news is that, by their very nature, autoantibodies (the cells that are attacking healthy tissue) come and go, creating an ideal backdrop for a "spontaneous remission" we can nudge along with healthy breathing and imagery.

3. *If receiving any kind of treatment, we want to imagine it being imminently effective.* This applies to nutritional supplements or anything else you're doing for your health. Such a simple suggestion is not to be overlooked because prior learning can get in the way. One woman had always believed that if she were ever diagnosed with cancer, she would choose some type of alternative medicine. When diagnosed with breast cancer, she surprised herself by electing to undergo treatment with traditional medicine. But to do so, she needed to overcome years of negative conditioning so that she could embrace chemotherapy as a healing agent.

This is accomplished not only through the skillful use of persuasive statistics, but also by tapping into the emotional center of the brain, the limbic system. If earlier conditioning is not in our best interest, imagery can open a door to new possibilities. When we discuss studies and other rational evidence, I'm speaking to the part of your brain that will determine whether or not to buy into what I'm saying. The evidence helps you decide, so I have to include a lot of it. But unless I'm telling you a really good story, the emotional center of the brain hears all my explanations as, "yadda, yadda, yadda." And yet this is the part we so desperately need to reach—where images are translated into a physical reality. This region, the limbic system, has 40 percent more neuropeptides (chemical messengers that can lock into immune cells) than the rest of the brain, and is the very heart and soul of the brain's emotional network. We want to work with and influence this part of the brain because your beliefs are formed here.

That's where the power of this technology comes in—by imagining a positive outcome you can overcome negative conditioning or lingering doubts and boost belief in your recovery while reducing potential side effects. A very petite seventy-year-old woman was scheduled to receive radiation therapy to her esophagus. Her doctor told her to expect to be very sick. Because she was already thin and frail, he was especially concerned that she would lose even more weight. But in her mind's eye she painted a yellow protective covering on the non-cancerous portions of her esophagus that the radiation couldn't penetrate. She had no pain and no difficulty swallowing after radiation; in fact, she gained two pounds during the course of treatment.

4. Considering that imagery works on the limbic level, it's easy to see why *it needs to be syntonic or harmonious with our beliefs.* If you are a devout pacifist, imagining an army of soldiers attacking your unhealthy cells is not congruent with your beliefs and could be stressful to mind and body. Personalized imagery resonates with the big picture as you see it, is rich in inner harmony, and connects the dots, as it were, to various aspects of yourself and your health.

This reminds me of Sylvia, an audacious woman with a recurrence of an aggressive type of lung cancer. When her doctor told her she had perhaps a year left to live, Sylvia immediately stood up, grabbed her purse and announced that she was going to buy a fabulous black dress. When the astonished doctor asked why, she snapped, "To wear to your funeral." She trounced out of the office, found a new doctor, and five years later, related that story to the group and me. Knowing her, it was no surprise that she chose to imagine her chemotherapy as a moving, twisting hose that was so powerful all of her body systems were cleansed in a matter of seconds.

5. To conclude your imagery, *you want to see yourself healthy, happy, and doing something you love.* This last step can release powerful will-to-live chemicals and create an association between being healthy and enjoying your life. Before I learned this essential ingredient, every time I imagined myself well I saw myself engaged in my work, which at the time was less than satisfying to me (i.e., this was not a rewarding image!). After learning to see myself creatively fulfilled, doing meaningful work, and spending time with people I cared about, my imagery took on new meaning. This isn't to say it has to be complicated. If you love snow skiing or lounging at the top of a mountain summit, and find that reminiscent of being vibrantly alive, it's valid. In addition to its physiological effects, this step can influence your mood, help you develop new possibilities and beliefs about your life, and give you a sense of control.

The story of Rick ties together all of the five steps. Rick was a single parent, thirty-two years old, with forty-five abdominal tumors. Experimental treatment at Memorial Sloan-Kettering had not been effective; he was given a morphine pump and sent home to "get his affairs in order." Rick did not want his four-year-old son to see him die at home or in a dreary place, so he came to Getting Well,[96] not because he thought he'd live but because he thought it would be a cheerful place to die. Even so, he willingly participated in imagery because it left him with a peaceful feeling—and because it was something he could do effectively while on morphine. Rick was a neatnik by nature. He was so fastidious, he pictured his white blood cells as vacuum cleaners operated by maids in sparkling uniforms, cleaning up all of the dust balls that symbolized the cancer cells. (This is a great image because a vacuum cleaner is much more powerful than a dust ball!) After he saw all of the cancer cells eliminated, maids with new vacuum cleaners were posted as sentries throughout his body for continuous protection. He then saw himself healthy, happy, and doing something he loves to do. Rick practiced this imagery at least three times a day. Over time he needed less and less morphine. The tumors began to shrink and three years later he was pronounced cancer-free.

In summary, Rick's imagery meets all of the five steps. It is uniquely his own, in harmony with who he is, and is playful but physiologically accurate. The metaphor for his white blood cells is more powerful than the symbol for the cancer cells, and he sees the cancer completely eliminated each and every time. His immune system is vigilant but balanced, and he concludes his imagery by seeing himself healthy and doing something he loves.

As you scroll through possible images for yourself, you don't have to worry about making a wrong choice. Your conscious mind can create lots of appealing imagery and symbols but, if they're not personally right for you, you won't be able to make it work. I often tell patients our job is to get out of the way. With practice, you'll learn to let your imagery just happen in accord with your intent, whether it's problem solving, healing, or personal development.

Even though you ultimately want to own the process, the Resource Guide includes some excellent sources for imagery CDs that are not only relaxing, but also help fine-tune the process. Emmett Miller, M.D., created a CD entitled *Healing Journey* that integrates the steps above in a soothing, dreamy way with the sound of the surf in the background. At a conference I was checking out several CDs to purchase for the cancer center and during a break I went back to my room to try *Healing Journey*. When I woke up I had missed the first thirty minutes of the afternoon lecture! Since I slept through the CD, I had to go back and listen to it again (wide awake this time) and make sure it was what we wanted. (Truth be told, I had to get a latté and a notepad to stay focused. Dr. Miller has a CD for insomnia but this is the only one I need.)

Unless you have someplace you need to be, falling asleep while listening isn't such a bad idea. If you've ever fallen asleep to the TV or the radio you know how your subconscious can integrate what you're hearing into your dreams. So even while dozing you'll still absorb the healing image, and it may even prompt some ideas of your own. (Just make sure the message is one you want.) If the CD gives you an image that isn't working, try using it as a launching pad for your own imagery or as an opportunity to explore an entirely new direction. Most importantly—don't force a fit. One beautiful CD has an image that interrupts my process every time. The woman's voice is deep and melodic, the music and sound effects are luxurious, and I can get quite relaxed. And then she mentions a healing blanket that creeps up my body (that's not how she puts it but that's how I hear it!) and no matter how deeply relaxed I am or how I steel myself to block out the image, as soon as it's mentioned I'm out of that nice zone and ultra alert, kicking off the blanket in my mind's eye. Yet plenty of others relate to the same image and find it soothing. It may be helpful to order a few CDs to try and then exchange with friends. Even though I most often rely on my own imagery, when I'm tired or not feeling up to par, it's refreshing to listen to somebody else tell me how to do it.

Imagery as Medicine

Like a daydream, the scene or image can take on a life of its own. Dr. Rita Joy Stucky of the Menninger Clinic (a pioneering center for the use of imagery) first opened my eyes to the full potential of imagery. While much of what she shared was enlightening, it was her own story that stopped me in my tracks and made me take stock of my own imagination in an entirely new way. When Rita developed severe eye pain and redness, she first chalked it up to all the hours spent knocking out her dissertation. But problems lingered and an ophthalmologist diagnosed scleritis, an autoimmune condition that attacks the sclera, the white part of the eye. If untreated, the condition commonly results in blindness. The doctor explained that there wasn't much they could do for her other than palliative care and offered Rita some topical steroid drops. After investigating the bleak prognosis, Rita decided to use imagery. She had been working at Menninger and explains, "We recognized at the time that the body's information comes to the conscious mind in the form of images. These images are representations or templates that hold the body's directions for creating and recreating everything in the body; including health and disease." Her clinical work showed that if you could get a clear intuitive image, "then you're working with the body directly and dramatic change can occur. The revolutionary idea for me was actually deciding to do for myself what was working with my patients." Becoming deeply relaxed and allowing the imagery to unfold before her she found herself standing next to a huge culvert. "In retrospect I know that it was a blood vessel, but it was colored a deep red and it felt very hot; too hot. Then it started to snow—cooling and insulating the vessel; and each snowflake represented a cell of the sclera replacing itself. Within a very short time my symptoms totally resolved. I never used the steroid drops. Twenty-three years later there is no problem with my vision."

Chest pain proved to be a warning sign to Robert, who immediately sought evaluation and was diagnosed with cardiomyopathy, a serious disease in which the heart muscle becomes inflamed and doesn't work very well. In his mind's eye he "visited" the area around his heart and found a ragged garden outside with a heavy fence between his heart and the garden. The fence pressed on his heart and felt too tight. Robert began by asking the fence how it was helping him. The fence made it clear that it was there for his own protection. Robert thanked the fence for all its good work, but asked if it would be okay if they made a little room for the heart. At first the fence resisted and Robert listened and again expressed appreciation for all that the fence had protected him from over the years. "But now we need to grow together. Even you need room for yourself and with a little healthy space you can keep protecting me." So the fence took a step or two back, and in doing so, changed color and shape, becoming something more pleasing, like a fence around a garden, rather than a menacing "No Trespassing" sort of fence. When that happened, the garden "seemed to need my attention, and so now I'm cultivating it."

When Richard started having prostate problems he was told that it was typical for a man of his age. Not willing to accept that entirely, he mentally "talked" with this area of his body and got a sense of "pebbles and stones" that were blocking "some tubular structures." He asked about the pebbles and got the sense that they were "old injuries," and so he said, "I reached in and plucked them out one by one."

While most of the interactive messages in imagery don't require immediate action, a sobering lesson taught me to deeply respect any warning given. Rachel had an inoperable brain tumor and was receiving radiation treatment. She held an image of a wizened Yoda-like creature sitting on top of the tumor. The creature didn't talk to Rachel, but would monitor the tumor, giving her signals of one sort or another that all was well. In her imagery, the tumor continued to shrink. It was a crisp fall day when Rachel came into see me—ordinarily the kind of day that would have her feeling ebullient. But she was visibly upset. The creature was now red in color and dying—the tumor nowhere to be found. "In my imagery I'm relieved to find that the tumor is gone, but I'm sorry to lose my little friend. It's as if he's absorbing the radiation meant for the tumor. I'm scheduled for a treatment this afternoon and a brain scan next week, so we'll see then if it really is gone."

After radiation, Rachel picked up her three-year old daughter at daycare and had a stroke driving home. She made it into her garage and managed to hit the emergency button on the alarm system before collapsing on the floor. Rachel's brain tumor was indeed gone; however, the radiation had also killed healthy tissue and caused bleeding in the brain.

With grit and grace, Rachel climbed back from her stroke and a dozen years later remains cancer-free. I share her story because if Rachel had insisted on a scan before having that last treatment, she might have been ridiculed—hospital staff could have given her a hard time—but considering the alternative it would be a small price to pay. So whether your image suggests a medical issue or implies further testing, follow through for peace of mind if nothing else.

Intellectual knowledge alone is not enough to create true healing. We must go beyond the logical, linear mind and reach our heart of hearts, a place of deep personal truth. Research indicates that relaxation and imagery can assist in recovering from trauma of almost any kind, whether from a shocking diagnosis or surgical procedure, an abusive childhood or the wounds of war.[97] (The Resource Guide can help connect you with professionals who have experience with imagery, but in general many clinical psychologists have experience with imagery and other helpful techniques.)

To develop your own image, establish an intention and gently ask for a representation of the problem along with its solution, and then relax. While some symbols arise spontaneously, others take several days. But what if you're repeatedly missing a key ingredient? Let's say that the sense of being joyfully and vibrantly alive just doesn't happen in your imagery. Don't worry or judge the experience, accept where you are in the process while considering the concept of joyful vitality. What memories are aroused? What might it take to feel like that again? Coaxing it out, you may play with the concept for a few days, gently cultivating and nurturing the possibility of feeling enthused about life. (A few other helpful tricks are in the Get Started Now exercise "Your Healing Image" at the conclusion of the chapter.)

There is a shortcut you can take advantage of, though. Since your brain automatically engages in problem-solving while you are sleeping, you can capitalize on this by asking for the image—or the solution to the problem—right before falling asleep. Then, when you first begin to wake up, while you are still in that dreamy state between deep sleep and wakefulness, you can explore any images that may be there.

Some people think of the subconscious as some spooky subterranean world—and it certainly can be that, especially if you're having bad dreams! But you may not realize how much it does for you in everyday life. Let's say you were discussing movies with someone at a dinner party and in the course of conversation were unable to recall the name of a well-known actor. Frustrated, you let it drop so the conversation can move forward, only to have the name suddenly pop into your mind on the drive home. That's a gift from your subconscious mind.

When we do things so often that they become second nature our conscious mind doesn't have to direct a lot of energy that way and the subconscious can take over. Imagine how much effort it took initially to learn to type. What if it took that much concentration every time you did it? Fortunately, we can type pretty much without thinking about it, which means it's happening on the subconscious level. Perhaps you need to be awake at a certain time, maybe earlier than usual. If you do, indeed, wake up at the time you wish, it's compliments of your subconscious, because your conscious mind was asleep! There are certain features of consciousness that defy explanation—such as your ability to return a fast moving tennis ball or baseball. Did you know that the ball can be moving at speeds of up to one hundred miles per hour? That's far faster than your conscious mind can track it![98]

Get Started Now: Your Healing Image

The following exercise introduces your healing image, but then becomes a guided imagery exercise that you may or may not choose to follow. See what happens as you go along. Feel free to use the script as a jumping off place and follow your own imagination from there. You can read all the way through and let yourself drift off into your own place of exploration, listen to it on my website, or easily make your own audiotape by reading into a tape recorder, making any changes you like. The sound of your own voice is meaningful to your subconscious mind.

Take a few deep breaths and exhale slowly. Begin again in your special healing space, the place you visited at the beginning of the chapter. Breathe in the aromas, feel the textures, and embrace the peaceful safety of this beautiful area. Notice if there are any changes or adjustments that you would like to make. Is there anything that would make this place even more comfortable? If it seems good to you, allow that to happen now and become even more relaxed in your safe and comfortable healing corner of the world. Let yourself linger in the peaceful solitude. When it feels right, with gentle attention, imagine a symbol for the problem you may be experiencing. It might be a physical challenge or a personal obstacle that needs your care.

Perhaps the problem has a color or a shape, a feeling or a sound. You may see the problem in your mind's eye or you may visit the place in your body where the problem resides. Notice any change in movement, shape, color, or size of the problem. The symbol may or may not appear, but you can trust and believe in yourself, knowing that you carry within you just what you need. You may choose to stay and observe for a while, but whenever it feels right, imagine the problem resolving in a way that makes sense to you. Perhaps there is a healing light or other force, maybe even a color, moving and soothing, releasing and refreshing. Feel your body coming into balance and harmony again. Be in your body now and feel the energy, all of your cells responding to your intent, releasing anything that might be in your way. Gently and lovingly cleanse your body and your mind, opening every cell to light, to love, and to healing. Feel the energy move throughout your body, balancing all of your organs and tissues, bones and muscles. Trust and know that this healing energy goes exactly where you need it the most. You can just relax and enjoy the sensations; you don't have to make anything happen.

Focus your attention now gently on your heart, bringing understanding and compassion wherever you need it most, including all aspects of your life. Take your time. When it feels appropriate, remember what it's like to feel vibrantly and fully alive, perhaps going back to a place in time when anything seemed possible. You might have felt joyful, peaceful, or excited. In your mind's eye, what is your posture like and how does it feel to be in your body? Moving confidently and joyfully, feel this special time of your life come alive. Bring the fullness of that experience into your body now and relish the sensation of strength and the feeling of hope as you open each cell in your body to light, to love, and to healing. Imagine again doing something that you love to do, bringing all your awareness to the moment, using all your senses to feel how good it is to enjoy completely. When you're ready, pat yourself on the back and congratulate yourself for participating in your recovery in such a meaningful way. And now, feeling deeply rested but energized and alert, gently bring your body back to the room, back to your awareness of space and time, back to where you are, and into the present moment.

Tuning in to Creative Problem Solving

Imagery can be done almost anywhere and your eyes do not necessarily have to be closed. You can just glance at your hands in your lap, with an easy sort of relaxed attention. When used deliberately and purposefully, it's a super way to decrease the wear and tear of stress on the body and fight the energy drain of suspicious symptoms and endless rounds of medical tests and procedures. Any opportunity for a healing interval will do. One woman practiced her imagery while parked in her car after dropping off and before picking up her children from school. (Never while driving, of course!) The more often you do it, the more fluid the process becomes. Many choose to do their imagery before falling asleep at night, programming the healing they want to occur while they sleep and again upon awakening. By adding a break during the day you'll give yourself an added dose of imagery and a relaxation session. Giving ourselves permission to take a few minutes a day to do this gives our body a "will to live" message and demonstrates that we matter to ourselves.

Imagery further reinforces health and wellness by changing the channel on worry, creating gratitude for the here-and-now, and bringing us back to the present moment with appreciation for all that is right within us. In this relaxed state, we are able to gain new insights as we turn down the volume on mindless chatter. When we do so, a fresh perspective on old problems emerges along with new opportunities and possibilities. What seemed like an endpoint becomes a turning point. We're more readily able to engage in the present and don't have to work so hard at letting go of the past or fretting about the future. A sense of majesty is born along with the ability to enjoy an enhanced perspective of the beauty and richness of everyday life, including the challenges and obstacles.

Perhaps most importantly, the regular practice of meditation, imagery, and relaxation results in peace of mind. After invasive procedures or treatments, and especially for chronic conditions, imagery can restore a sense of tranquility and well-being. There is a pragmatic side to all of this as well. Imagery and relaxation offer us precious moments to interrupt all the busyness and tune in to what our bodies really need. Our culture is oriented toward the quick fix. If we have a headache, we take an aspirin. When tired, we drink coffee. If tense, we have a gin and tonic or a tub of Ben & Jerry's Cherry Garcia. Becoming deeply relaxed and acutely aware of what our bodies need allows us to respond in a more appropriate and healing way to our bodies' requests. Imagery, with its power to evoke significant physical responses, becomes a tool we can use to examine which behaviors induce tension or relaxation, rob or create energy, and constrict arteries or relax heart muscles. Imagining the outcome of a choice through imagery is a rich method of connecting with our personal truth as we learn to be our own healer. Making a decision regarding treatment, where to live, or which job to take, can become easier as the right choice becomes quickly apparent when we tune into how our body reacts to each imagined alternative.

Changing Channels in Your Brain

But that's not all. The electrical currents or signals flowing through our bodies interact with our environment and exert an effect in any given moment in time—on our hearts, our brains, our muscles, and even the walls of our cells. This vibratory and electrical energy can be measured, such as with either an EKG, which measures the electrical rhythm of your heart, or an EMG, which measures the current in your muscles. Likewise, an EEG (electroencephalogram) is a portrait of the electrical signals of your brain. If you've seen brain wave rhythms in action you know that they vary in pace and pattern. Rapid brain waves called beta occur when you're engaged in a thoughtful activity such as balancing your checkbook or reading some challenging material. Slower alpha waves appear when imagining yourself in your beautiful scene like you did earlier in the chapter. If you can recall a time when becoming drowsy while reading, and your arm dropped along with the book—that was theta, an even slower rhythm often mistaken for sleep. And finally, it's the deep, restorative rhythms of delta that signal the familiar state of true sleep.

We can slip in and out of these states sometimes with annoying rapidity, as you know if you've ever felt sleepy in the middle of a conversation or lecture. In Philadelphia I worked for an innovative company called Advanced Neuroscience, where brainwaves were monitored as relaxation training took place. Our medical director, Dr. Carl Sonder, and clinical supervisor, Janet Eggen, taught patients to sustain a theta state for fifteen minutes twice a day using a customized relaxation tape at home. Long-standing problems of anxiety and depression were alleviated and I saw many people benefit.[99] For our purposes, alpha and theta rhythms are linked to states of healing and repair on a variety of levels. Every time you engage in imagery you're likely entering these restorative states!

Helping you do so are the properties of music and sound. While music is pleasurable and adds a rich dimension to most any experience, it has healing properties all its own. The next chapter will lead us into the electrical and vibratory nature of our cells and show us ways we can use sound and music as medicine.

ℰᕫ

WHITE BLOOD CELLS: THE BACKBONE
OF YOUR IMMUNE SYSTEM

There are many different kinds of white blood cells with just as many different functions, but their overriding mission is to keep you free from dangerous toxins, harmful pathogens, and cancer cells when they arise. The ways in which they protect you are miraculously diverse and not unlike some of the stylized, special effects in superhero action movies. In this case, these superheroes are protecting you! Your *natural killer* cells, for one, are like silent assassins, seeking out and vaporizing cancer cells, viruses and other harmful invaders. *Phagocytes* swoop in and devour foreign cells and substances. Videos of phagocytes in action look like the suction arm of a vacuum cleaner as they morph into action, reaching out and sucking up unwelcome invaders. *Neutrophils* are phagocytes that are like kamikaze pilots, entering the infected area to gobble up as much as they can and then dying themselves in the valiant act of saving you. (When you have a wound that forms pus, these neutrophils make up that yucky substance.) Like storm troopers, *Monocytes* can leave the bloodstream, enter the tissues, and swell up to five times their size. In their large size they are called *macrophages* and they have multifaceted superhero abilities. When defending healthy tissue, they can squirt specialized enzymes into invader cells or act as scavengers and gobble up debris. At other times they may secrete a bleach-like agent to destroy foreign cells. If they are unable to completely destroy an organism, they may encapsulate it, keeping it separate from the body. And like something from a *Star Trek* series, they can even fuse together and form giant cells. Sometimes white blood cells sniff out invader cells in a process called chemotaxis. Other cells can protect you by releasing histamine when attacked by toxins or bacteria. The net effect is a walling off of the affected area from surrounding tissue, which minimizes the spread of infection.

Week Three

❧ 5 ❧

Good Vibrations: Music and Sound as Medicine

Music gives flight to the imagination and soul to the universe.

—PLATO

Music has power to affect even the deaf. Symphony solo percussionist Eveyln Glennie performs with major symphonies throughout the world and cannot hear a sound. Evelyn learns new compositions by hugging a stereo speaker or holding a cassette player and tunes her instrument, the tympani, by feeling the vibrations in her face and feet. Through touch and the sensation of sound she has learned to "hear" music.

Simply put, sound is energy. Sonic abilities help bats and dolphins navigate and oceanographers map the slopes, ridges, and trenches of the ocean floor. Sound even has a direct effect on solid matter, as when an operatic diva hits just the right note, and matching the natural frequency of the glass, shatters a crystal goblet. Sound waves engineered with exquisite precision target and pulverize kidney stones in one hundred thousand patients every year. The very first photos we have of our children often come our way compliments of ultrasound technology, which produces detailed pictures of developing babies small enough to fit into a tablespoon. Sound can also have deadly consequences. In the Austrian and Italian Alps during World War I, the power of sound brought fifty thousand soldiers to their deaths as the sound waves created by their gunfire triggered catastrophic avalanches.

Our interest in sound isn't new. Chants, dirges, lamentations, and songs of praise were integral parts of everyday life in ancient cultures. In fact, we have yet to discover a human culture that doesn't have music.[100] Even today in most rural African communities, call and response singing is still practiced as it has been for thousands of years. That tradition became a beacon of hope and promise for slaves in America because, encoded in the chant—a hymn of the underground railroad called "Follow the Drinking Gourd"—were instructions for finding the North Star, hence the way to the North for slaves willing to risk their lives for freedom.

From freedom trails to avalanches, the effects of sound are far-reaching. But when we think of sound, we most often think of music. In Europe, before Bach could wow us with his fugues and cantatas, a written code for musical notation was needed. While ancient Greece and Rome had a written system for documenting musical notes, that knowledge came to a crushing conclusion after the fall of the Roman Empire, as it simply disappeared during the Dark Ages and was lost to the medieval world.[101] The church of that time frowned on musical instruments—for their use in pagan culture and for the distraction they caused—but chanting was permitted, first without real harmony or rhythm, and later a cappella harmony was added, followed by instruments.

The rediscovery and reinvention of musical instruments took some strange turns. While a hydraulic organ from the third century BC could be played with a light touch, early medieval organs were so massive that organists played by banging with their fists on levers some five inches wide and a foot long; these organs were fed by hundreds of pipes, with dozens of men on huge bellows.[102] It was said that the townspeople trembled and shuddered in the presence of such sound.

From those humble beginnings, Gregorian chants were eventually notated and a code gradually emerged over the centuries to form what would become the musical transcription we have today. Increasingly sophisticated, now we can measure the effects those rhythms and tones have on our heart rate, our breathing, our brain waves, our immune cells, and even our DNA.[103] What we know puts music and sound squarely in the middle of any modern day pharmacopoeia. Endorsing that idea medical oncologist Mitchell Gaynor, M.D., writes that sound "...should become part of every healer's medicine bag."[104] In this chapter you will see how you can quickly and easily incorporate the stunning physics of sound into your own medicine bag of healing technologies.

A stone is frozen music, frozen sound.

—PYTHAGORAS, GREEK PHILOSOPHER (SIXTH CENTURY BC)

Just What the Doctor Ordered

As Evelyn Glennie proves, there's more to music than meets the ear.

Frequency (the rate of vibration) is one of the most important elements of sound and one of the fundamental components of energy. In medicine, sound is commonly used as a diagnostic aid. If you've ever gone for an ultrasound or an echocardiogram, then you've experienced sound waves bouncing off organs and tissues, the vibrations creating patterns that are recorded for a radiologist to read and interpret. Whether the picture was of a fetus or of the chambers of your heart, it is a product of sound.

Correspondingly, our cells (and even some viruses) are impacted by frequency or vibrational patterns, either positively or negatively. New research shows that cell membranes (now understood to be the "brain" of the cell, rather than the nucleus) rely on certain vibrational patterns and disturbing their healthy movement can give rise to disease.[105] Just as an operatic high note shatters crystal, vibrations "can deactivate a number of viruses," according to Arizona State University physicist Kong-Thon Tsen. In the last two years, eight of his peer-reviewed studies demonstrate that vibrations of a certain frequency can explode the outer shell of the virus. Using a special laser, his most recent work destroyed HIV in test tubes.[106]

Deforia Lane, Ph.D., knows better than most the power of music and sound to heal. A teacher, therapist, opera singer, and twenty-five-year breast cancer survivor, Dr. Lane was the first music therapist to receive a grant from the American Cancer Society to study the effects of music on cancer patients. Currently, as the resident director of music therapy at the University Hospitals of Cleveland Ireland Cancer Center, her work has captured the heart and attention of health professionals across the globe. But for the children who fill the beds at the Cleveland Cancer Center, music does more than comfort and inspire. In a novel experiment, Lane successfully demonstrated that a single session of music therapy could boost immunity in hospitalized children. Reported in the *Journal of Oncology Management*, a measure of immunity (salivary IgA, an antibody naturally occurring in our saliva) was significantly increased when pediatric patients were exposed to as little as thirty minutes of music therapy.[107]

How We Know: Sonic Bloom

Numerous investigations have demonstrated music's ability to enhance our well-being on multiple levels.[108] Some of the research has a razzle-dazzle quality to it. In her book *Positive Energy*, psychiatrist and author Judith Orloff, M.D., writes, "in monasteries where monks play Mozart to animals, the cows give more milk; with critical-care patients, classical music has proved just as relaxing as Valium; fetuses have preferences, too—they settle down hearing Vivaldi, but rock music agitates, causing violent kicking."[109] Other studies have established that music can help you awaken from anesthesia sooner and with less pain and can serve as a general analgesic if you happen to live with chronic pain. It can also help normalize cortisol levels, boost endorphins (feel-good chemicals), augment your relaxation practice, and even affect your DNA (more about that coming up). Further studies demonstrate that, for those receiving cancer treatment, music therapy promoted relaxation and reduced anxiety,[110] which comes with its own benefit package.

Music helps plants grow, drives our neighbors to distraction, lulls children to sleep and marches men to war.

—DON CAMPBELL, AUTHOR OF *THE MOZART EFFECT*[113]

Further evidence comes from a 2008 study published online in the medical journal *Brain*, demonstrating that listening to music in the early stages following a stroke can improve recovery. In this eye opening study, sixty stroke patients were divided into three groups: a music group, an audio book group, and a control group. For two months the music group selected music they enjoyed and the language group chose audio books to listen to, while the control group did neither. Follow up evaluations revealed that verbal memory improved 60 percent in the music group, 18 percent in the audio book group, and 29 percent in the non-listening control group. The music group saw other improvements as well, such as less depression and the ability to focus and resolve conflicts.[111] Supporting these findings, a study of cardiac rehabilitation patients found listening to music while exercising increased scores on a verbal fluency test. For this investigation, scientists at Ohio State University specifically chose patients with coronary artery disease because the condition can affect cognitive ability. While most patients felt better after exercise, with or without music, the group that exercised while listening to Vivaldi's *Four Seasons* had more than double the improvement in verbal fluency than the non-music group![112]

Plants, too, respond to music—or more specifically perhaps, vibration. Fascinating studies have shown that certain sounds stimulate plants to grow faster while other sounds such as hard rock cause them to wither and die. One agricultural pioneer found that even poor, malnourished plants could thrive when exposed to nature sounds like birds and crickets.[114] Intrigued by numerous studies in Europe suggesting that classical music could stimulate plant growth, Carlo Cignozzi thought it just might help his grapes. Cignozzi has a vineyard in Tuscany and after wiring his vineyard for sound he noticed that the grapes weren't only growing faster, but they were healthier, too, free of molds and fungus. The music even served as pest control, scaring away critters that would normally feast upon his grapes. As news of his success spread to the press, scientists at the University of Florence became formally involved—and are now sipping a little wine along with their research. Preliminary results show that the music—or its frequency—is working as Cignozzi hoped.[115]

The Pied Piper

It so happens that frequency has an intriguing side effect. Remember the fable about the Pied Piper? He didn't know it at the time, but the rats could have been following him because of a phenomenon of physics known as entrainment. Birds flying in formation and fish swimming in unison in schools are capitalizing on this facet of synchronized rhythm. According to the experts, the effect is universal and the physics extend to our own physiology, and powerfully so. A Dutch scientist, Christian Huygens, discovered in the late 1600s that if several pendulum clocks were mounted on the same wall, they would very quickly bring each other into perfect synchronicity. Each pendulum begins oscillating in harmony with the others, until they move as a single entity.[116] Likewise, muscle cells from the heart, pulsing independently of each other, begin to beat in perfect time when they are moved close together but do not touch.[117]

This phenomenon is one possible explanation for music's effect on heart rate. The most common objection, though, to using music to influence heart rate and blood pressure is that they can be fickle measures, changing throughout the day for a variety of reasons and when shown to be beneficial, sometimes the changes are small and not long lasting. But there is deep and practical evidence for utilizing this low-key intervention. A case in point is a study of patients who had recent heart attacks. Those in the music group had significant reductions in heart rate, respiratory rate, and heart oxygen demands. They were also found to have an increase in heart rate variability, one of the best measures of predicting survival after a heart attack.[118] Overall trends show that exposure to steady noise and certain types of music such as hard rock, techno, or rap increase arterial pressure, while listening to something personally enjoyable can lower these measures.[119]

Additional research bears this out. Dr. Karen Allen, research scientist at the University of Buffalo's Department of Medicine, measured blood pressure and heart rate in twenty people one week before surgery for cataracts or glaucoma, and then again on the morning of the operation, and every five minutes throughout the postoperative period. In all patients, heart rate and blood pressure shot up the day of the procedure, but in the group that listened to music of their choice (with headphones before, during, and after surgery), their "cardiovascular stress dropped significantly…within ten minutes of tuning in and remained low. …Only in the music group did cardiovascular measures nearly reach baseline."[120]

Taking Control

Pied pipers aside, unless we're selecting a CD, we may not consciously consider sound very often. As we wrangle our way through traffic, dodging honking drivers and sirens, we interface with a world of beeping pagers, cellular ring tones, chirping faxes, and email alerts, before settling down in front of two hundred television channels delivered by satellite directly to our living rooms. While we're surrounded by sound waves, from microwaves to radio broadcasts, we often take the energy of sound for granted.

But what you don't know you're hearing *can* hurt you. Researchers at the University of Chicago evaluated subjects' blood sugar levels while plying them with subtle sounds during sleep. None of the soft noise was enough to wake anyone up but it was enough to decrease subjects' ability to regulate blood sugar by a whopping 25 percent. Just three nights of poor sleep is the blood sugar equivalent of gaining twenty to thirty pounds, enough to predispose them, over time, to type II diabetes.[121] Although currently underutilized by most patients, major cancer research centers, such as Memorial Sloan-Kettering and The University of Texas M.D. Anderson Cancer Center, routinely incorporate music into traditional protocols.[122] Europe, however, leads the way and has been the most progressive in the regular use of music therapy as an adjunct in cancer care and compromised immune systems. In Norway alone, there are over two hundred "music baths" in use where the body is "bathed" in sound and vibration.[123]

There is good reason to offer music, as the constant bleeps, buzzes, and signals we're subjected to in hospitals have been shown to induce anxiety.[124] Becoming aware of what we hear around us, including background noise, can be crucial when healing, and we need to be aware when sound blocking becomes a necessity.[125] One study showed the simple use of headphones cancelled out the cacophony of the hospital setting, reducing anxiety in the process. Since most hospitals aren't yet taking advantage of this low-cost, highly effective technique, it makes sense for family and friends to help you out if you're suddenly hospitalized—or come prepared if you know of your hospitalization ahead of time. By selecting your own music, you can easily create and customize more supportive rhythms to entrain or synchronize with than hospital noises.

During hospitalization and surgical procedures, music and sound offer an opportunity for patients to take control and minimize feelings of vulnerability, reduce feelings of restriction and confinement, and assist them in reestablishing a sense of personal power. When you're feeling vulnerable, music offers a visceral escape. One woman said music accomplished that for her when she created a "cocoon of sound that became its own sweet reward."

Of course individual differences in taste are important. Musically accomplished individuals, such as pianists and composers, can find it difficult to practice imagery or relax deeply with some music because it can be a distraction rather than a help. In that case, some of the people I've worked with prefer ocean, nature, and abstract sounds. Respect your preferences and go with what feels right to you.

Like Grace, whom you met in the last chapter, you may want to consider using music if you happen to need surgery. Zeev Kain, M.D., of Yale School of Medicine became curious about the documented effect of music reducing the amount of sedation required during surgery. He wondered if music simply served as a sound blocking technique—muting the clanging and banging noises common in surgical suites—that accounted for the results. So, in a controlled test either white noise or music of the patients' choosing was filtered into the operating room during surgery. The outcome? Only the music group showed a significant drop in the amount of sedative required![126]

If you have advance notice of surgery, with your surgeon's permission spend time before the procedure imagining an optimal outcome while listening to a specific composition. Then, as agreed upon ahead of time, play the CD during the operation. Follow-up studies are strong, showing that along with imagery, the practice can even reduce postoperative pain.[127] As a result, some hospitals are using music consciously and intentionally for the good of the patient—and their bottom line.

(The Resource Guide has options for prerecorded imagery and music for surgery.)

Research notwithstanding, much about music's effects remains mysterious. Celebrated neurologist and author Oliver Sacks recounts how some patients with Parkinson's disease may be "unable to walk, but can dance perfectly well, and others although unable to speak a simple sentence, are able to sing songs verse by verse."[128] In a randomized trial of thirty-two Parkinson's patients, weekly sessions of music therapy were helpful in reducing the slow movements that characterize the disorder.[129] In a recent conversation, psychologist and author Kathleen Brehony reminded me of country singer Mel Tillis, who stutters like crazy when he speaks but can sing without a hitch. Even patients in comas have experienced dramatic recoveries and changes in consciousness when stimulated by music.

The Nature of Sound

Defining sound, Robert Tusler, professor emeritus of music at UCLA, explains that it's an "energy that can be reproduced into shapes, patterns, figures, and mathematical proportions, as well as into music, speech ... [sound] goes directly into all our body systems and unfailingly triggers reactions, conscious and unconscious."[130] Tusler's words came back to me when I was standing in a subway terminal and noticed a display of photographs of the most beautiful crystalline shapes I had ever seen. At first I imagined they were magnified snowflakes. But they weren't. What I was admiring were the effects that words, emotions, and music had on water! Captured by Japanese researcher Dr. Masaru Emoto in a unique photographic process, classical music produced beautiful, symmetrical crystals while heavy metal music yielded distinctly distorted asymmetrical shapes.[131] Considering our bodies are roughly 70 percent water, it makes sense to carefully choose the words we say (or sing) to ourselves and the sounds we surround ourselves with—especially when healing, when everything matters.

As mesmerizing as the physics of sound are, we don't have to entirely comprehend the effects to take advantage of them. Since background noise can influence our physiology, we can scrutinize our own environment for sounds we might have become accustomed to. Imagine the implications of the University of Chicago study that found subtle night noises significantly reduced participants' ability to regulate blood sugar. (You may not consciously register the clock chiming midnight or your snoring partner, but your health may suffer.) For solutions try the Sound Survey, parts I and II.

Get Started Now: Sound Survey Part I

Now that you understand the effect sound waves can have, you can take advantage of the principles in your everyday life by first becoming aware of the sounds in your environment—background noise included—and the effect they have on your mood or heart rate. In this first part of the survey, you're playing sound detective—not necessarily coming to conclusions or making changes—you're just taking notes on what you find. You might want to start by jotting down how you choose to wake up in the morning. What sounds do you begin your day with? After you're up and around, is the TV on or is it quiet except for noises from the street? On your way to work notice the sounds of traffic and what you usually tune into on the radio. In a sound-conscious way move through your day, making note of typical sounds and noises, noticing how each one feels. Be sure to include an estimate of how many times your cell phone rings (or vibrates—remember sound is vibration) and the bells and whistles on your computer or the PA system. Follow the trail of sound up until bedtime and then during the night. Obviously, you don't have to wake yourself up to do this, just take note of typical nighttime sounds such as a snoring spouse, a teenager's music, or the sounds of sirens from the street.

One client of mine is a dentist. When we first talked about this exercise, he immediately thought of all the drills and noise-making equipment that are the heart and soul of his profession. Rather than dismiss the exercise out of hand, he pursued it and discovered several discretionary sources of sound: talk radio on his drive to the office, the televisions in each exam room often tuned to news channel CNN, background phones ringing from the front desk, conversation between employees, music in the hallway and waiting room, cell phone calls from family and friends during lunch, sirens and talk radio on the way home, squabbling siblings and kitchen sounds, television, the chime of a grandfather clock, and finally, the alarm at 5:00 a.m.

You can see what he decided to do about certain aspects of the survey in part II, but for now, take stock of the sounds in your own environment.

An antidote to noise pollution was conceived by sound artist Bruce Odland. Judith Orloff, M.D., in *Positive Energy*, writes about her interview with the artist: "Commissioned by the city of West Hollywood, he installed a 'tuning tube' on the sheriff's station, which, he explained, 'makes a beautiful harmonic out of chaotic traffic noise.' The result? A humming, chanting, and a soothing wah-wah...Along that stretch of sidewalk, this human-friendly sound helps nullify squealing brakes and honking horns. I hear from the locals that pedestrians practically rejoice in relief. They report feeling happier, get along better; some have even broken into dance and song."[132]

Yet sonic or vibrational intrusion isn't necessarily limited to what we can hear. ELF waves and Electromagnetic Fields can have an effect on our own energy and cell wave frequency.[133] Controversy over the safety of radio signals from cell phones prompted the European Union to launch a four-year study (titled REFLEX) investigating the effects. While emphasizing the DNA damage is inconsistent and not necessarily harmful, and reminding the public "there's no reason to panic," the recommendation is that landlines rather than mobile phones be used whenever possible. Ronald Herberman, the director of the University of Pittsburgh Cancer Institute says that although the evidence is still controversial, he recommends, "Children should only use cell phones in emergencies."[134] Some neurosurgeons, including Dr. Sunjay Gupta, CNN's medical correspondent, use an earpiece to keep the microwave antenna away from their brains. It's not that these technologies are necessarily "bad" for us, but we want to take a close look at what they are accomplishing for us or what they might be depriving us of.

In part II of the sound survey, I ask folks to take a deeper look at the cumulative toll of all the beeps and buzzes of our plugged-in world. At first people tell me that it's not a bother, that they enjoy being tuned in to everything and everyone around them. And that may be true, to a degree. Our multi-techno-colored world didn't just suddenly appear, though. If it had, we might have registered effects we've become desensitized to. Instead, like the frog in a pot of cool water that doesn't leap out even as the water heats up, we've incorporated each new device into the fabric of our lives without taking stock of the total effect.

I knew I had fallen into the "frog in the pot" habituation trap when some colleagues came to stay with me for a while. My answering machine was on as usual, my pager was in my purse, and my cell phone in my car (which made me think I was really in control of technology). After a few days they exclaimed, "How can you stand it? We don't know how you can get any work done, there's so many interruptions, and for heaven's sake turn off the volume on your answering machine!"

My buddies happen to be pioneering researchers at a major university. I knew for a fact that they were taking advantage of technology on a daily basis. But they recognized the intrinsic value of uninterrupted quiet as a prerequisite for reflection and creative work. (How much more so when accomplishing the all-important work of healing!) I got the message and took a second look at my own sound survey with fresh eyes—or ears I should say. There's no denying that connectedness is important, but it's possible to stay in touch without being "ding-donged half to death," as a friend of mine describes it.

Untangling our technological umbilical cords can be liberating, as our group discussions show. One participant, whose cell phone was connected to her hip, relegated it to the car for "emergency use only," and signed up for voicemail through the internet so there would be only one messaging center—her computer—to check daily for either voice mail or email. She checks just once a day despite complaints from family and friends. She gets more done with fewer interruptions and has reclaimed her quiet space for much needed enrichment. "I'm still available and connected to all the people I care about—but just not every second of every day. When I'm with friends who haven't taken the sound survey, I realize how unnatural and nerve wracking it is to be at everyone's beck and call. Even call waiting keeps you from connecting uninterruptedly." Technology is a tool. Take the sound surveys and look for ways to keep it in its place.

Get Started Now: Sound Survey Part II

Now that you're aware of the many sources of sound in your environment, you can begin consciously choosing how to use sound to your advantage. The first step is to identify which sounds are beyond your control and which ones might be under your influence, marking your list with a plus or minus sign.

Let's look at the list of sounds over which you have no control. In the example of the dentist, he included on his list: dental equipment, sirens, conversation, television in the exam rooms (chosen by the patient), background phone ringing, waiting room sounds, and squabbling. He lowered the volume on the phones at the front desk and coordinated the waiting room sound (formerly tuned to a news station) with that of the hallway, choosing music for both. With the open exam room style of the practice, there wasn't much he could do about conversation except install white noise speakers in strategic areas, which provided some relief. But what about the televisions in the exam rooms? It seemed everyone wanted to watch CNN's *Headline News*. The innovative solution here was to tell people they might feel more relaxed with some music. The TV was tuned to a music channel and each patient was offered a headset with several musical selections. Not everyone chose music though. A fair number still wanted a news channel, but when working with those who did choose the music, the dentist and his staff got bit of a break. For his drive home in Atlanta (where traffic is reputed to be among the heaviest in the nation, second only to Los Angeles), he consciously considered the effect he wanted to create for himself in his car and selected his music accordingly.

As for sirens, Kathleen Brehony's solution is the most soulful. Whenever she hears a siren she told me she says a prayer for the person or the situation. It reminds me of agape, the Greek word for love based on principle. This kind and loving energy is a reminder of our collective humanity, displayed by compassion to strangers. Kathleen's graceful response transforms a stressful sound into an opportunity for connection and reflection.

Get resourceful with your solutions, brainstorm ideas with friends: perhaps a pair of ear plugs to block street noise or your snoring spouse, a small bubbling fountain in your cubicle, a white noise producer for the waiting room, lowering the volume on all the ring tones in your environment, turning your cell phone off except for the precise times you want to be available to callers, and telling the children to squabble someplace else.

There's so much we can't control that we especially want to pay close attention to what we can. Take a good hard look at the sounds marked with a plus sign, the ones you do have control over, and consider each one carefully. Capture the cumulative effect of the complete picture, fully grasping the effect on your energy, mood, and sense of well-being. Continue to notice how these various sounds are affecting you. For a short cut, you can use your "gut" to feel your way through your options, reviewing in your imagination the physical effects of each one. It might mean waking up to a favorite piece of music or a CD of ocean sounds rather than the clanging alarm clock. The morning news might be minimized, or on the drive to the office, you might choose a happier vibe than talk radio. When cooking dinner, ask yourself if you really want the TV on or if listening to a Puccini opera might feel more festive. Identify your choices and then choose consciously.

Psychoacoustics

A few years ago, a defense attorney from Atlanta sat in my office, telling me about all the cases piling up on her desk, her anxiety about leaving home in the mornings, and the lengths she would go to avoid eating in public. Three months prior, she had been fine. But one afternoon, when eating a candy bar in the office of a colleague, she looked down and noticed half of a roach was in the next bite. The next thing she knew, she was unable to converse, or look up from her plate, and she couldn't stop cutting up her food into tiny little pieces. She wouldn't eat away from her home and the anxiety and social isolation were affecting her job performance.

Everyone has a threshold, a limit to their psychological "space," the point where we become aware that we may not be coping as well as we were in the past. That threshold is different for each one of us and when crossed requires different strategies for repair. We all know "stress hardy" folks who ride the roller coaster of change without a care or a whimper. Others are more sensitive, and as multiple traumas and life changes pile up, it can be the seemingly small trigger that unravels the sense of wellbeing we've so carefully crafted.

The attorney had seen a psychiatrist and received some much-needed medication, but the patient wanted to augment the prescription with some behavioral medicine strategies, and so the psychiatrist referred her to me. Of the techniques we explored, it was the technology of psychoacoustics that helped her the most. After a few weeks of using a headset and a special CD twice a day, she was not only back in the courtroom, eating with colleagues and friends, but off all medication.

Combining research from the fields of psychology, physiology, and acoustics, psychoacoustics is the study of the perception of sound. While some evidence reveals only minor benefits, other studies report improvement in many conditions, including depression and anxiety. A 2001 study of people with mild anxiety reported marked improvement when using a psychoacoustic tape once daily for four weeks.[135] Prior to that, researchers at Duke University found the technology effective in staying alert for certain tasks.[136] More recently and perhaps most importantly, psychoacoustics has been found to significantly decrease presurgery anxiety—which affects outcome.[137]

The centerpiece of this technology is the binaural beat. Using ordinary headphones along with a specially made CD, a listener hears a different beat in each ear, which causes the brain to form a phantom beat.[138] This third frequency, known as a binaural beat, is the difference between the two incoming frequencies. The brain responds by raising or lowering brain waves to match it. Electroencephalogram (EEG) results show that the binaural beat can produce a corresponding change in the brain wave rhythms themselves—possibly due to entrainment and resonance.[139] Brain wave rhythms, like sound rhythms, are measured in cycles per second, and each state is associated with different mental and emotional characteristics. It could be increased concentration (beta), healing (theta), or deep sleep (delta), depending on your goal. (See the previous chapter for more.)

This integrative science has emerged from the robust research of at least two institutes of sound. One of these is The Monroe Institute,[140] which for the last twenty-five years has been a leader in researching and evaluating the effects of different sound patterns on mental states, including those that are inaudible to the human ear. The second cornerstone of sound research comes to us from the Tomatis Institute. French physician Alfred Tomatis, an ear, nose, and throat specialist, spent decades studying hearing, and developed techniques that achieved astonishing results with autistic children. Using high frequency recordings of voice, Gregorian chants, and Mozart, Dr. Tomatis prescribes sound as a means of strengthening and rebuilding neuronal activity in the brain for those who have learning disabilities, depression, chronic fatigue, and other immune disorders.[141] (The Tomatis Method has also received recognition among abuse survivors as a gentle yet effective technique for working through and moving beyond trauma.)

Other perks include increased concentration, better memory, stronger language skills, wider vocal range, and greater clarity of hearing. If you shop around for CDs with this technology, you'll find several designed for health that include guided imagery along with the psychoacoustics. (See the Resource Guide for a selection.) In my experience, psychoacoustics doesn't automatically lock listeners into a certain brain wave rhythm, but it can give them a nudge in that direction and offer some support in maintaining that state for a therapeutic length of time, especially if the listener is distracted or particularly antsy. As your mind wanders, the gentle rhythm and sounds can bring you back to your healing image. (Keep in mind that simply closing your eyes and imagining yourself at the beach changes brain wave rhythms, too.) For a psychoacoustical CD to be effective, hearing a different beat in each ear is essential, so listening with headphones is a must. This may be one reason why the attorney mentioned previously found it effective—headphones can create an inner oasis of peace—and two, the binaural beat may have helped her sustain a theta rhythm for a period of time, allowing her neurotransmitters to come into balance.

Overall, any relaxing or enjoyable music can facilitate imagery, making it easier, more pleasurable, and providing healthy perks along the way. Studies by imagery pioneer Jeanne Achterberg and music therapist Mark Rider show that sound used synergistically with imagery gives an added effect of reducing stress hormones and boosting immune cells.[142] And if you'd like to feel a bit sharper mentally, one recent study reported that listening to any music you find enjoyable can boost cognition, while another found listening to Mozart raised students' IQ scores by a few points.[143]

Your Healing Voice

Technology aside, the qualities of your own voice can change the vibrational pattern in your body to support and strengthen healing. A French composer and bioenergeticist, Fabien Maman, teamed up with Helene Grimal, a biologist at the French National Center for Scientific Research in Paris, and using microscopic photography, documented the effect of low frequency sound (thirty-forty decibels) on human cells.

Mitchell Gaynor, M.D., writes, "Using a camera mounted on a microscope, Maman and Grimal studied the inner structure of both healthy human cells and uterine cancer cells as they reacted to various acoustical instruments, e.g., gong, xylophone, acoustic guitar, and the unaccompanied human voice, for a duration of twenty-one minutes.

"Maman found that the most visibly dramatic results occurred when he sang musical scales into the [cancer] cells: 'The structure disorganized extremely quickly. The human voice carries something in its vibration that makes it more powerful than any musical instrument: consciousness...but the other instruments, particularly the gong with its rich complement of overtones, also caused the [cancer] cells to disintegrate and ultimately explode." [144]

You've experienced the vibrational pattern of your own voice whenever you have instinctively hummed to yourself or perhaps, when feeling heartbroken, allowed a low keening sound to come to the surface. Some of these more primal sounds, like wailing or laughter, seem to bubble up and explode with surprising force, and we feel better later for it. Have you ever been in a serious meeting, gotten tickled about something, and tried to stifle your giggles? The energy needs to escape, so you might have been shaking a bit in your seat (more embarrassingly, you might even snort). Worse yet, try and control a wail.

I was reading about these findings when I first met the mouse in my cabin. The next thing I knew, I was—like Olive Oyl—standing on top of the little gingham loveseat screaming my head off. He made a rapid retreat—for about a minute. He was a bold soul, peering out at me from beneath the kitchen cabinets or peaking around the corner of my wastebasket. We'd lock eyes and I would bang on something or make another loud noise, but nothing seemed to faze Mickey except an earnest and energetic yell.

As you might guess, I'm not really into bugs or rodents, but I didn't want to harm the little guy. I also knew the effect of all those stress hormones, so I baited a couple of "be kind" traps with some peanut butter, but he wasn't falling for it. He was totally on to me: racing by the traps, tripping the door, laughing I'm sure. But only screaming would make him hide. Determined to relax, I imagined him as Ratatouille, the mouse chef in the animated film, but I still didn't want to see him gnawing on the furniture, so I'd give a good holler, as they say in the South.

After two weeks of this, it was hard to muster up anything like my initial fright—the honest enthusiasm required for good screaming—so I'd lounge on the sofa, relaxed and almost content—and just start yelling. What I noticed was that no matter how relaxed I was, my heart would begin racing as soon as I started screaming. Even if I screamed while stretched out like a cat, the effect was the same. My remote location insured that no one would call 911, so I was free to continue experimenting, going for effect with pots and pans, claps and whistles, but it was the sound of *my* scream in *my* ears that did it every time—heart pounding—pulse over a hundred beats a minute. (After hearing about all the noisemaking going on, my husband was feeling sorry for the mouse!)

Clearly I was changing the vibrations in my body. The noises we make, happy humming, weeping or wailing—or screaming as the case may be—have a physical effect. If screaming while relaxed could send my pulse racing, then why not the reverse—a calming sound perhaps? It turns out to be true, but fortunately other experiments are a lot more sophisticated. Dr. Gaynor reports laboratory findings of experiments with two breast cancer patients who used their own voice in a technique called *toning* for three and a half hours a day for one month. In one woman the tumor simply disappeared. In the other, surgeons found the tumor was "reduced and completely dry and she made a full recovery."[145]

Toning reminds me of a deep resonant hum that vibrates throughout the body. Focusing more on vowel sounds, but including any natural sound that emerges, the idea is to echo or mirror the natural "hum" of your body and then follow the wave of sound as it changes. The crux of the theory is that vocalizing sounds changes the vibration of the body.

With what scientists are unlocking about the vibrational patterns of our cells, frequency is key to healing on a cellular level. Some clinicians and physicians are using this idea to stimulate the body's own healing mechanism. This may not be as farfetched as it sounds. Or maybe it gets even weirder. Geneticist Susumu Ohno of the Beckman Research Institute in California converted genetic equations into music. Each of the four basic nucleic acids was assigned two consecutive musical notes and was composed into an exact duplicate of the genetic code. For example, when translated this way a segment of mouse RNA (similar to DNA) became music when played on the piano: specifically, a portion of Frederic Chopin's *Nocturne*.[146] Since all our cells possess a "tone," the vibration isn't a one-way street.

On another note (forgive the pun), neurologist Barry Bittman, M.D., of the Mind-Body Wellness Center in Meadville, PA, has found that playful music-making can reverse the stress response on a cellular level, positively affect immune function, reduce burnout, and improve mood. Atlanta physician Judith Chiger, M.D., is on the bandwagon, so to speak. She brought her collection of Health Rhythm drums and tambourines to the cancer center so we could experience the full effect as we tapped, toned, banged, and jingled our way to feeling more relaxed. Most of us can tap a drum and shake a tambourine, so performance anxiety isn't a threat and each individual is free to express his or her own rhythm, even within the group.

It all sounds like good fun, but Dr. Bittman's findings on the genomic impact of recreational music playing are especially telling. He explained to me that any stressor that influences the body affects us on the genomic or DNA level, long before our blood pressure goes up or our hands become ice cold. In the first phase of one of his studies, researchers induced stress by asking participants who didn't enjoy jigsaw puzzles to put together complex ones. Folks then either played music or put their feet up and read magazines or the paper. Of the genes that were expressed, three times as many were reversed with the recreational music-making as opposed to a typical mode of relaxation, such as reading the news.[147] (It would be great to see a similar comparison with imagery and music.) Backed by Yamaha, Dr. Bittman is waiting on the results of the genomic impact of acute stress followed by music-making on eighteen thousand functional genes in individuals facing the challenges of heart disease. Stay tuned for the outcome.

Other health practitioners demonstrate our ability to resonate or oscillate to a particular frequency by using tuning forks to align the body's "sound" to a healthier level. President and Medical Director of the Alzheimer's Research and Prevention Foundation in Tucson, Arizona, Dr. Dharma Khalsa uses sound to speed healing from brain injuries or cognitive decline associated with dementia or even carbon monoxide poisoning.[148] In patients with Alzheimer's, a four-week music trial (listening in the mornings for thirty or forty minutes) increased melatonin levels significantly. Melatonin is a naturally occurring hormone that can help regulate circadian rhythms; researchers report that it could be one reason that participants in the study were more relaxed and calm. Best of all, the result still held true at their six-week follow-up.[149]

Mood Music

Music goes further than the rat-a-tat-tat of studies, technology, treatments, and techniques, beyond the dazzling display of physics, anecdotes, and case studies—and straight into our hearts. Music can make us weep with joy or wail with grief, accompany us on a road trip to get away from it all, or take us back to a time we want to remember, when anything seemed possible. From the soaring symphonies of Hayden and Vivaldi, to strains heard in places of worship and places of play, music is evocative of memory, time, and emotion, able to raise us out of a dungeon of despair or release tears like much-needed rain in a dry desert.

Music's redolent power isn't new. Ancient Greek philosophers believed that music possessed moral character. In *The Republic*, Plato states that music is much more powerful than the laws of society and that the wrong kind of music produced undesirable character traits, while good music produced noble traits in the listener.[150] Aristotle believed that music affected behavior and reflected the passions or states of the soul, such as anger, hope, or courage. Pat Cook, founder and director of the Open Ear Center for Music in Healing in Washington State, writes that Pythagoras prescribed daily singing to cleanse emotions of worry, sorrow, and fear and "Musician-physicians composed melodies to cure passions of the psyche, as well as depression and anger."[151] And long before the Greek civilization became a world power, David soothed King Saul with compositions on the harp.

As you might guess, listening to music involves the limbic system, the part of your brain responsible for emotion. Most researchers agree that this area of the brain is also responsible for intuitive leaps of insight and creative problem-solving ability—something we want more of when facing any kind of trial or crisis. It is easy to imagine the sheer panic of receiving a life-threatening diagnosis. In this anxious state, little productive problem solving takes place. Techniques that help us reestablish control and reduce anxiety greatly assist in improving our ability to make decisions, which can literally be a life-or-death matter.

Years ago it seemed coincidental when someone mentioned to me that they had stopped listening to music before they got sick. Now, when working with patients I often ask, "When did you first stop listening to music?" Some answer immediately, having wondered about it themselves; others have to think for a week or two, but eventually most everyone puts their finger on the answer and realizes that, prior to the diagnosis, at some point they stopped listening to their favorite music. Adding it back mindfully can be beneficial. With music we don't have to work quite so hard—it creates a break in the wall. And sometimes music can do something for us we can't do for ourselves.

It reminds me of Greg, a classical pianist trained at Julliard who eventually left the stress and pressures of performing for a quieter life with his wife and twin daughters. A few years later, Greg's garden variety of non-specific symptoms and his feeling of ennui sparked his physician to prescribe a common antidepressant. At first Greg felt a bit more energized, but gradually the effect wore off and the medication was changed. The pattern continued over the course of three or four years until Greg had worked his way through several drugs with negligible benefits and unhappy side effects. His physician referred him to me, thinking that behavioral medicine might be an option. After discussing mind-body interactions and giving him time to practice diaphragmatic breathing, we talked about music. He missed it. Greg didn't miss performing, but with the pressures of being self-employed and supporting a family, music was relegated to a tiny corner of his life. Greg did some brainstorming and carved out twenty minutes each morning to play the piano. Over the course of two or three months he made other adjustments as well and no longer needs antidepressants.

Another way music can enhance your personal healing repertoire is through the isomoodic principle. This technique is based on matching music to an individual's current mood and then gradually changing the music to achieve a different emotional state, with physical benefits, too. While some types of music have been studied more than others, what really matters is how music feels to you personally and culturally. So explore a variety of music and sound and then consciously choose based on your intuitive wisdom or gut feeling in that moment. Ask yourself if you want to be soothed, comforted, and nourished or stimulated and revitalized? If feeling frayed, do you need release or renewal? Are you resonating with soft, nurturing tones, floating meditative ones, or music that is energizing and vibrant? Focus on your intent and how you feel physically, and match the sound for the desired effect.

Get Started Now: Choosing Good Vibrations

Now that you've begun cleansing your acoustical world, you can choose to add sound for a specific effect depending on your intention. You may want to start by experimenting with the isomoodic principle. First notice how you're feeling now. Take a look at your iPod or your CD collection and choose a piece or two that reflects that feeling. For the sake of illustration, let's imagine that you happen to be feeling wistful or bittersweet. You might choose Pachelbel's *Canon in D* and see if it resonates with your feelings. If so, spend a few moments exploring in a non-judgmental way whatever comes up. From this place, decide how you would like to shift your mood. Perhaps your intent is to move into a more vibrant, passionate state. If so, you might try Vivaldi's *Four Seasons* and see how you feel when "Spring" is being played.

Browse through your musical selections or download new selections, choosing certain pieces for driving time, cooking, cleaning, or doing chores. Experiment with sounds of nature or abstract combinations if you're engaged in something creative. If your heart is racing, notice how it feels to listen to something that has sixty beats a minute, like some Baroque pieces or soothing ocean sounds. If you've been feeling a bit "under the weather," try listening to Mozart, Vivaldi, or another Baroque artist for twenty minutes twice a day. If you enjoy the process, explore the exercises presented by Don Campbell in his book *The Mozart Effect*.[152] They're interesting, fun, and designed to heighten our awareness of the effect that music has on us—mentally, physically, and emotionally.

Singing along with your favorite music can be invigorating—and good for you. While healing, folks often choose the music of their teenage years to relive the feelings of indestructibility and the sense that anything is possible. Donna Jenkins is forty-five and has beaten breast cancer on not one, not two, but on three separate occasions. Most recently cancer cells were found in her brain and the side effects from treatment left her dizzy and her gait unstable, and she was unable to drive. As she recovered for the third time, she wanted to take a trip away from the February drizzle to sunny California, where she grew up. And she wanted to drive! Her husband rented a convertible and she and her two daughters drove up and down the California coast singing along with the Rolling Stones, Joe Cocker, and the Steve Miller band, the music of Donna's youth. She came home grinning, feeling lighter, younger, and freer. Music can form a bridge between our perspective of life before the illness and the perspective we hold after. Singing, like toning, can release energy and nurture and support neglected parts of ourselves.

Music that offers exquisite beauty while instilling a sense of safety and support, combined with pieces that inspire, can become an integral part of the healing process. In the six-week class, I encourage everyone to make their own personal music tapes or collect CDs for various circumstances and changing moods. A collection of music ranging from pieces to empower, relax, help conquer fear, release tears, and provide comfort is a practical tool during the emotional and physical recovery after illness or a diagnosis.

If you are part of a group or would like to start one, music can be part of the package. At ECaP (Exceptional Cancer Patients), when celebrating or sharing meals, one of our team, Clinical Social Worker Sally Baumer, would choose upbeat music from different eras, such as big band music, a soft jazz collection, or an invigorating Latin vibe. If a group is newly formed, or during a brief retreat, music that brings people together—such as simple chants, sing-alongs, or folk tunes—sets the tone. When concluding a health retreat at ECaP in which the members have tightly bonded and are going back to distant areas of the world, the group forms a circle, holds hands, and sings a lovely chant from *On Wings of Song*, "Listen, listen, listen to my heart song/I will never forget you/I will never forsake you."

By now you understand that various states of consciousness produced by thoughts, intentions, imagery, and sound, have a frequency—a vibration—that affects us on the cellular level. Using music to create moments of solitude, reflection, and imagery, as well as bathing the body in the rhythm of entrainment, contributes to physical and emotional rejuvenation while enriching our experience. Continue to look for ways to incorporate music and sound into your own healing program. It is an enjoyable way to make a difference in your health and improve the quality of your life.

In the next chapter you'll discover the power of resonance and meet someone whose life was saved by a mariachi band. (And if you're wondering about the mouse, I installed a couple of sound frequency devices—inaudible to people, but not to mice. It took a couple of days, but I haven't seen him since.)

৵ 6 ৵

Creating Resonance:
Harnessing Energy for Healing

If we really want to live, we'd better start at once to try; If we don't it doesn't matter, but we'd better start to die.

—W.H. AUDEN

If you deliberately plan to be less than you are capable of being, then I warn you that you'll be deeply unhappy for the rest of your life.

—ABRAHAM MASLOW

You could hear a pin drop in the auditorium. Every seat in the house was taken. Physicians, therapists, and clinicians sat riveted as Marion Woodman, Jungian analyst, international lecturer, and acclaimed author told her story. Widespread metastatic cancer had depleted her energy and finally her will to live. She described it as being behind a curtain or veil—on one side were all the activities and emotions associated with living, while she existed on the other side, remote and disengaged from life. As fatigue and apathy continued to overtake her, she was not uncomfortable but quite content to let life slip by, and in time she stopped fighting the process of dying.

While she was in this state of mind, some friends insisted that she and her husband attend a large party. Marion reluctantly agreed. After a couple of hours, tired and somewhat bored, she signaled her husband that it was time to leave. Just as she did so, a mariachi band came marching through the room they were in. Marion said, "I felt the music move through me and my body remembered what it was like to be young and healthy. I turned to my husband and said, 'Let's dance.'" He replied, "But Marion, you can't," yet she insisted and they danced. In that very instant Marion discovered that the veil had lifted between life and death and she found herself wanting to belong once again to the world of the living. And there she was before us—strong, radiant, and cancer-free. It was an unforgettable moment for all of us.

Healing requires the ability to engage fully with life. It can happen in a flash or stem from painstaking and deliberate effort. Regardless, there is no more potent immune stimulant than the will to live. Being actively engaged with life involves more than just living longer, counting off the days in months or years, existing, as one woman put it, "in God's waiting room." A member of our group at the cancer center loves to illustrate that point with the following story: A man was diagnosed with a life-threatening disease and told he had just six months to live. "But doctor, isn't there anything I can do?" asked the man. "Well, yes, there is, as a matter of fact. First you can buy a pig farm, the biggest one you can afford. Then you can marry a widow with eight children, ages four to seventeen." "And then I will be cured?" "No," replied the doctor, "but you'll live the longest six months of your life." The idea, of course, isn't just to prolong life, but to fill it with zest and meaning. Cancer specialist Gerry Goldklang is convinced that the neurochemical process engendered by the will to live is so extraordinary that it is unmatched by any pharmaceutical. The by-product can include beating the odds.

We can begin to exploit this natural pharmacy and gain another edge over the odds by understanding the factors that cause some people to live longer than expected. There are three factors, but only one of them has an exceptional effect on your longevity. The first is the fear of dying, which can extend life a bit longer all by itself. The second is staying alive for someone else, such as seeing a child through high school or helping a dependent mate gain certain skills. But the strongest factor that can profoundly lengthen life is when our own passion for living—for life and all it has to offer—is so grand that the immune system is influenced in a statistically remarkable way. Living fully, regardless of test results, often reflects an inner state of congruence or harmony, a reflection of how in tune we are with our deepest nature. To do this requires that we know ourselves in more than a superficial way.

How We Know: Teasing Out Resonance

Teacher and psychotherapist David Lee likens the mind-body relationship to an orchestra and symphony. The mind and body are two different things, but intricately connected. If the room is too cold or the musicians are in a bad mood, the orchestra will affect the symphony. On the other hand, if the musicians are inspired and the audience is connected, the outcome on the symphony can be grand. When all parts of a system are in tune, operating in a healthy, creative, and energetic state, we call it resonance.

We know from high school science that the universe is all about vibration and that resonance is not simply a concept, but a dynamic of physics. It can be demonstrated by using a guitar and a piano. If the E note is played on a piano, the E string on a guitar will vibrate, even if the guitar is on the other side of the room. In our "see and touch" reality, the physics of resonance provides the seeds for miracles, for it can be experienced within our bodies in much the same way as in the guitar and piano. When our emotions, passions, and intellect are in tune, dissonance disappears, energetic blocks are erased, and the unity produces a dynamic engagement with life.

When we have resonance, our perspective, our innate positive qualities, and our performance are amplified in all areas of our life in a domino effect. "Once, after listening to several of his lectures, a newspaper reporter asked the wife of Mohandas Gandhi, 'How is it that Gandhi is able to speak so interestingly without ever repeating or contradicting himself even though he uses no notes?' Mrs. Gandhi replied, 'Well, you and I, we think one thing, say another, and do a third—but for Gandhi they're all the same.'"[153]

If what we think, say, do, and feel are unified, the harmonious image gives rise to resonance, whereas an incongruent pattern creates dissonance within our bodies. Cultivating resonance is not as mysterious as it may seem; in fact, it can be surprisingly simple. Perhaps you recall the story of Mark, who had salivary gland cancer. Although he was given only six months to live, he is healthy and cancer-free now many years later. Although he never considered himself the creative type, one way he pursued the challenge of his cancer was through art. He felt he needed to do something he had never really done before, that wasn't related to job or family. So rather than jumping straight into the work day as soon as he awoke, he changed his schedule. Each morning he would put on some music and quietly do the drawing exercises from Betty Edwards' book *Drawing on the Right Side of the Brain*.[154] (Creative work and recreation enhance certain skills that relate to problem solving.) In addition, he practiced imagery and relaxation exercises. This led to positive changes at his place of employment and eventually to an improved relationship with his wife and children. Soon, there was more of a congruent and integrated pattern to his way of being and relating to himself, his work, and his family.

Get Started Now: The Five Things

The approach below has a cumulative effect. Even if you aren't certain of your answers, simply asking yourself the questions opens your heart and mind for an

"Aha!" experience that can occur when you least expect it. To begin, get a pen and paper and try the following:

After becoming relaxed, focus intently on what you love to do. Through the lens of your imagination, allow yourself to capture moments of zest, inspiration, or pleasure. Take your time. What is your posture like? How does it feel to be in your body now? Do not limit yourself; select as many life-enhancing activities or moments as you like.

Now notice what sort of moments or activities left you depleted, spent, exhausted, or simply apathetic and bored. Feel fully the effect of these. Allow yourself to experience any muscle tension or change in your posture or sense of well-being. Note the contrast to feelings of being reenergized, revitalized, or simply refreshed.

Next write down at least five things you love to do (whether or not you actually do them) and five things that you do not enjoy doing. Hold on to this list and we'll take a look at it soon.

One of the best ways of determining what you love is to notice what makes you lose track of time. Work, study, play? Over the next couple of weeks, stop every few hours during the day and notice how you feel. Acknowledge energy draining activities—how do you feel before, during, after? Pay attention to your thoughts. This is not an exercise to establish how you believe you are supposed to feel, but how you really feel; what are your symptoms—or your energy level—telling you?

The Coin of Your Life

As we noted in Mark and Marion's stories, your physical body responds readily to resonant messages through clear, dynamic energy. When our emotions and intellect are divided, though, the resulting conflict can bring on physical symptoms. Psychotherapist and founder of Getting Well Deirdre Brigham calls this phenomenon the "morality of the body."[155] Unfulfilled potential and stifled dreams first "kill the spirit and then the soul," according to the grandfather of mind-body medicine, Dr. Lawrence LeShan.[156] The solution, he suggests, is to pay close attention, and by doing so we will be in a position to begin moving the priorities of our lives to the front burner. Simply being willing to do the exercise above creates an

Time is the coin of your life. It is the only coin you have, and only you can determine how it will be spent. Be careful lest you let other people spend it for you.

—CARL SANDBURG

opportunity for a shift to occur by letting your subconscious know that you intend to create a life that is personally meaningful and joyful for you.

It reminds me of Sisyphus, the mythological Greek who, as punishment from Zeus, was compelled to roll a gigantic boulder uphill that would just roll down again, over and over. If our daily life resembles that of Sisyphus, then our health may be in jeopardy. In a study at the University of Texas over two thousand people were polled in a national survey that assessed general health, physical function, and how they spent time. They were asked about their work, volunteer projects, and whether they had an opportunity to learn new things or do something they really enjoyed. The overwhelming finding was that creative activity— defined as non-routine, enjoyable, with built-in learning and problem-solving possibilities—helped people stay healthier and live longer. The lead author of the study, Professor of Sociology John Mirowsky, found that creative work can have a biological effect of causing the body to appear nearly seven years younger than chronological age![157] Upgrading the quality of our lives means learning new things, being challenged, and participating in enjoyable creative activities. (In a later chapter we'll see how many centenarians fit this overall profile.)

All of which is challenged when we lose touch with what we authentically enjoy. Long-standing patterns may require a fresh perspective. Fortunately, we may have at least a little more control than poor Sisyphus.

Not long ago I was invited to present a workshop on "Living Well," and as a group we completed the exercise above (the five things). As the audience shared items on their lists, one man proudly stated that there was nothing on his agenda that he didn't like to do. Ever since retirement he did just what he liked and nothing more. I was wondering how this could even be possible when a woman on the opposite side of the room said she had only things she didn't like to do on her list. She added that she couldn't even tell me what she liked to do since it had been so long that she had had any choice in the matter. I jokingly replied that the two of them must be married to each other—and they were! (The room was crowded and they had taken the only seats they could find).

Developing a high degree of personal choice in the way we do things or how we live depends on accurate self-knowledge. To jump-start the discovery process, one physician asks his patients to remember what they loved to do when they were ten years old. Going back that far can provide seeds for rediscovery. To nourish your progress, keep a journal of activities and note how each activity or social setting makes you feel. Keeping a diary or reflecting on your day in the evening is a way to systematically take stock of the various influences on your moods, energy, or symptoms. Rate the effect of every endeavor, encounter, or experience on a scale of one to ten, with one being the least rewarding and ten being the most. (Watch your associates: some clinicians speak of emotional contagion—negativity can be contagious!)

After it is clear which items inspire the high points of your day, look for ways to increase the frequency of the positive experiences and decrease others. If some unpleasant activities are essential and ultimately unavoidable, don't worry. In chapter 8, you'll learn a trick for dealing with them, but for now, the goal is to become sensitized to how you really feel. Once you are exquisitely aware, you can begin making choices that better support your true nature. This cost/benefit analysis alerts us to how we've been using our physical resources so we can shuttle more energy into healing and repair.

The Energy Pie

When energy is consumed by adapting to change or coping with anxiety-provoking situations, less is available for keeping the body healthy. As we learned in chapter 3, over time the continued strain of unrelenting stress can deteriorate tissues and vital organs. To see where we can reclaim energy, in this week of the program, I draw a large circle on the board to represent "the energy pie."

The supreme accomplishment is to blur the line between work and play.

—ARNOLD TOYNBEE

Get Started Now: Your Energy Pie

Draw a large circle on a piece of paper and divide up the pie into the various activities of your life. The morning activities, such as getting ready for the day, usually take up quite a bit of space. Work, whether at home or outside the home, usually consumes a larger portion of the pie. Remember to include errands, laundry, or household repairs. Add any relaxation, watching TV, or walking the dog. And now we have grocery shopping, paper work, bill paying, phone calls, cooking, cleaning, spending time with family, etc. Notice how full your pie really is!

Imagine now that you have to work overtime. Waking up the next day you might be somewhat fatigued, in which case you begin that day having a little less pie because you borrowed from it to work late. Let's say after coming home from work that day you have an argument with your spouse and toss and turn most of the night. Now you have even borrowed into the following day's energy. By the time the weekend rolls around, how do you think you are going to feel? Will Saturday be a day of refreshment or will you need to just catch up from the energy drain of your week?

If we draw energy from further into the future, the body loses its ability to recover and we can become vulnerable to getting sick. When an illness develops, the energy pie becomes even more relevant as a portion of vital energy each day will be required just to heal. There is a silver lining though: certain activities actually generate energy. You've experienced a few of these already—abdominal breathing, deep relaxation, and music—that reinstate and fortify your energy. Rounding out the picture is time spent with people you love, laughter and play, exercise, music, art, and doing things that inspire or that you truly enjoy, all of which help restore lagging energy reserves.

Identifying insidious or hidden energy zappers—people, places, things, and activities—can help revive depleted energy. When one of my patients checks her social calendar, she says she does it, "looking for more pie." She deletes situations and people from her schedule that are likely to rob her of energy and adds activities and people that are mutually beneficial and refreshing. Paying attention to your energy pie helps you focus on the choices you are making and enhances your natural ability to heal while creating a more enjoyable life in the process.

Another way to look at it is that energy, like money, is a finite commodity. The effort and challenge involved in creating more energy is similar to saving and investing your money wisely. If funds have been depleted and you are depending on credit cards for basic expenditures, those items come with a high interest rate. Eventually, if you keep spending at the same rate, a day of reckoning will occur, in which case, careful scrutiny of income and expenses, checks and balances can help you formulate a plan to avoid bankruptcy. As debt is paid off you may then begin saving and earning interest on the money. Now it can benefit you—whether you save for the proverbial rainy day, travel somewhere fabulous, or take an online class at a university.

Reclaiming Your Energy

Until there's a surplus, our energy may solely go toward correcting the deficit that has accumulated. For many this involves extreme self-care, establishing a solid relationship with a health care provider, making sound dietary choices, and spending more time resting and sleeping. Sleep is a powerful anti-inflammatory and since inflammation is at the heart and soul of disease, at least one of the physicians I work with dispenses advice like "sleep more" on his prescription pad. A friend of mine, Ray Hill, deals with a cluster of complex autoimmune issues and emphasizes that, "No matter what I do, if I don't get the sleep I need nothing works." For him sleep is the linchpin for a host of self-care strategies.

Your brain needs sleep for other reasons. It's actually very active while you're slumbering away, oblivious to everything. Scientists now believe that sleeping helps your brain reorganize all the information that you've been exposed to during the day. Researchers in Germany uncovered evidence that the brain works on unresolved problems while we sleep, leading to spontaneous solutions the next day. (This may be one reason dreams frequently feature whatever we're concerned about.) And according to a recent investigation led by neuroscientist Dr. William Fishbein, sleep is critical to memory making.[158] But there are even stronger reasons to get your zzzs.[159] As it turns out, your body's ability to secrete growth hormone—an essential ingredient for repair—can be negatively affected by sleep deprivation.[160] It can even impact our mental health. Brain scans show that missing as little as a single night's sleep disrupts the part of the brain that keeps our emotional selves in check.[161] (Yikes!) Your body's hormone balance also depends on circadian rhythm, so getting into a steady sleep pattern is essential.[162]

Ideally, we should all just hit the sack and sleep until we're relatively caught up. When one woman tried this, she thought she'd lose her job, her friends, and her boyfriend because she slept so much. But she kept at it and once her sleep deficit was satisfied she settled into a nine-hour-per-night pattern that has her feeling fine. The beauty of the method is that the true amount of sleep you need as an adult will (eventually!) emerge and your optimal wake/sleep pattern along with it. During this time of repaying our energy debts and allowing our bodies to heal, it's vital that we have compassion for ourselves. Every illness requires a period of convalescence, a time of recovery when the body regains its strength and health. The word *convalescence* comes from the Latin and implies growing strong. One source suggests it originates from a Roman army bugle call that when played meant to regroup and then move forward. True convalescence will take time, thus it calls on compassion for yourself as you gain strength by "regrouping and moving forward," Rather than berating yourself or comparing yourself to others, treat yourself as you would a precious child who had fallen ill or a beloved pet that was injured. Soon you will have "energy dollars" that you can spend. Best of all, some of these expenditures can actually become investments, giving you even more energy.

The process is personal. Linda worked full time and rarely missed work even though she had been on chemotherapy for two years straight. Although she always appeared tired, she rarely complained. Then one week she seemed a little more animated and shared that she had hired someone to clean her house every two weeks. Her husband argued that it would be too expensive and that they couldn't afford it, but Linda pointed out that golf was expensive, too. (Her husband, an avid golfer, never said another word.) Linda admitted that it was not as clean as when she did it herself, but now she had Saturdays available to do things she loved and to create more energy for herself.

In one of my six-week classes, every participant had cancer except for one woman. Sandra Powers was there on behalf of her son, who was unable to attend. At twenty-two he was diagnosed with third stage Hodgkins disease and had moved back in with his parents. During the class Sandra took a lot of notes but was very quiet. When discussing the energy pie, though, I pushed her to share with the group. She spoke softly but distinctly about her full time job, another part time job she worked into her schedule on evenings and weekends, and caring for her adult son; her mother, who was handicapped and lived alone; and her mother-in-law, who was ill. Both of these women depended on Sandra to bring them their meals, deliver medication, take them to their doctor appointments, and run their households. Sandra had also been baby-sitting for her grandchildren on Saturday evenings and Sunday afternoons. But recently, all Sandra could think about was whether her son would live or die. The room was quiet. No one knew what to say.

The following week I asked the group if they had any thoughts or comments they wanted to share on our discussion of last week's energy pie. Sandra tentatively raised her hand and began to tell us what she had done. First, she called Meals on Wheels and arranged for meals to be delivered to both housebound women under her care. Next, she contacted the pharmacies closest to each and transferred prescriptions so that all medication would be delivered to both her mother and mother-in-law. She then called each of her adult children and told them that they were not to drop off their children without an invitation to do so or without making arrangements ahead of time. Even though finances were tight, Sandra spoke to the manager of her part-time job and reduced her overall workload. She accomplished all this in only one week.

The group wondered how all of these people had taken the tremendous change in their circumstances. "Oh, they were really upset and my mother and mother-in-law were downright nasty. Everyone tried to make me feel guilty. Both 'mothers' accused me of being a bad daughter while my children accused me of being a bad grandmother. It's caused quite a bit of commotion, I assure you." How, I asked Sandra, was she able to make the choice to stand up to all of that? "I went home and looked long and hard at my energy pie. I knew that soon there would be nobody to take care of any of these people if something were to happen to me. I had to 'love my neighbor AS myself.' If I don't care enough about myself to treat myself right how can I really do best by my family? And if they don't or won't acknowledge my life as being worth something, then I can't help them and wouldn't want to die for them. I want to live and I want to be around for my son's recovery. And by the way, I had my first Saturday off in ten years and it was wonderful. I even called one of my granddaughters to share it with me." That was over twelve years ago. I recently caught up with Sandra—she is healthy and enjoying life and her son has been cancer free for over a decade.

Fatigue Fighters: Fascination and Purpose

Sometimes what we think we want in life is not a personal desire at all but reflects the expectations of other people. This lack of emotional awareness can result in being isolated from ourselves. One woman in her early fifties stated, "I have operated in the realm of expected behavior for so long I honestly cannot tell you what I—as an individual—want." For some of us, the last time we thought about any of this was when we were teenagers. Things change—circumstances and people change—and it may be time for a refresher course on "you."

What strikes me is the fact that in our society, art has become something which is related only to objects and not to individuals, or to life. That art is something which is specialized or done by experts who are artists. But couldn't everyone's life become a work of art? Why should the lamp or the house be an art object, but not our life?

—MICHEL FOUCAULT

You may not have taken a personality assessment quiz since you were a teenager, but now is a great opportunity to fine tune what you know about yourself. The Keirsey Temperament Scale[163] (based on the Meyer's Briggs personality typing) cuts through years of conditioning and brings to light who you are underneath, whether you were raised by farmers in Idaho or artists in San Francisco. To give you an idea of how this might be helpful, there are common misconceptions about the traits of introversion and extroversion. You may be surprised to know that there are lots of entertaining and socially adept folks who are introverts—they just happen to refuel and restore their energy by spending time alone—while extroverts regenerate by being around other people. Just imagine how much energy you might be losing if you're an introvert who rarely has any alone time! Spouses and friends often enjoy taking the Keirsey and comparing notes; it can smooth communication and facilitate understanding and acceptance of fundamental differences. (See the Resource Guide for more.)

Answering this one question, "What do I want out of life so that I can experience more joy, enthusiasm, and zest?" is good medicine, although the answers may change with time. If our situation has changed it may be time to rediscover ourselves and make a direct inquiry as to what fascinates us now. When I was a teenager and young adult, the rougher the travel the better. I backpacked in grizzly bear territory and slept on trains across Europe (and in plenty of airport terminals) with eager enthusiasm. As time went by, though, that sort of travel lost a little of its luster and I came to expect a hot shower and a soft pillow. Years later, when I started complaining about a scary bed-and-breakfast I found myself staying in, my husband brought me to attention by reminding that there was a time when I stuffed socks in the holes of the walls of my room in Rome. (I wanted to make sure nothing crawled through, but I stayed on quite happily.) My perspective had definitely changed!

Since happy people are healthier and happiness is a predictor of longevity (more about this coming up), then it behooves us to notice what leads to happiness. It requires tremendous honesty to examine our lives, to distinguish between something that may make us materially comfortable but emotionally miserable. A labor and delivery nurse for thirty years, Gloria loved every minute of it until the last two years. "It no longer had the same pull it once did and I found myself feeling tired and not quite right." Recognizing that our emotional hooks get in the way of achieving our goals, the solution lies in cultivating awareness. Mihaly Csikszentmihalyi (Dr. C, I presume), professor of psychology at the University of Chicago, has spent the last twenty-six years investigating the state of passionate preoccupation he terms "flow," the sensation that athletes and dancers feel when their minds and bodies operate in total harmony, or when writers and artists lose themselves in their work and time seems to stand still. He found that flow generally occurs when a person is doing his or her favorite activity—gardening, listening to music, bowling, cooking a good meal, driving, talking to friends, and often working.[164] Very rarely do people report flow in passive leisure activities such as watching TV. During flow, our minds work at optimum efficiency, which makes us feel happy, motivated, creative, and in control.

We are all faced with magnificent opportunities, brilliantly disguised as impossible situations.

—AUTHOR UNKNOWN

Without it, we find it hard to focus and feel dissatisfied and bored with what we are doing.

A high degree of choice, concentration, and enjoyment of work is necessary to keep energy at a high level. Having a passionate pursuit—sport, hobby, activity, or interest—rekindles excitement and adds immeasurable zest to life (not to mention pie!). Not surprisingly, two of the most effective antidotes for fatigue are fascination and purpose. Immersing yourself in a network of intriguing possibilities keeps your mind charged with stimulating new ideas that spark joy. Get greedy—not for things—but for experiences! Dr. LeShan asks workshop participants to identify the "part of you that has never flown emotionally, physically, creatively, experientially."

Simply becoming aware of our true nature helps reshape our priorities. Suppose you have a hot coal in your hand that you are not even aware of. If something brings it to your attention, you don't have to be told to drop it, nor do you need special courage to do so. The response is automatic. With awareness, we can openly and honestly process any inner conflict that has sabotaged our peace and ability to heal. As barriers to happiness are removed (such as fears that restrict your life or unexpressed anger that is silently eroding a relationship), you will be defining and developing a congruency of thought, desire, and action that creates resonance throughout your body.

Building a Bridge to the Future

Courageously facing any conflict that arises, whether or not a solution is in sight, captures energy lost in dissonance and nourishes strong, personal reasons for living. This deep self-understanding demands an accounting of how we would most like to live the hours, days, weeks, and years that may be ours. If we refuse to acknowledge our mortality, we will lack this discernment in the mistaken belief that we always have tomorrow. Accepting our own mortality opens the door to resonance by helping us refine our choices about how we want to live today or what we would like to accomplish tomorrow. Imagine what an extraordinary life we would have if we accepted our mortality and engaged with it to create each and every year as the best year of our life!

When faced with difficult choices, I try to apply that mindset. When a producer for the *Oprah* show was interviewing me for a segment, he asked if I subscribed to the "live each day as if it were your last" philosophy. While I appreciate the principle, it hasn't helped me with day-to-day decision-making. (I answered that I wouldn't have spent the day before the film crew arrived vacuuming my house if I thought it was my last day of living!) I find it much more useful to ask myself what choices I would make if this were the last *year* of my life.

By way of example, about three years ago I was offered a wonderful opportunity. Soon after accepting it, I began to feel uneasy and more than a little irritable, so I reflected more deeply on my decision. It certainly seemed sound and I could find no real flaw in accepting the offer; in fact, it made perfect sense. So I asked myself if I would consider the position as time well spent if I knew I would be killed in an automobile accident a year from now. (It may sound extreme, but it often clarifies my bottom line position.) At that moment I knew immediately that I would deeply regret using my time in that particular way. And so, although it was rather last minute, I backed out. When I later chose another project to commit to and asked myself the same question, I had no dissonance whatsoever.

Some might say that they already have so many demands on their time that they cannot afford to do anything new or interesting. But more often than not, time stress is an excuse for not taking control of one's life. As the historian E.P. Thompson noted, even in the most oppressive decades of the Industrial Revolution, when workers slaved away for sixty to eighty hours a week, some spent the few free moments they had engaging in literary pursuits or scientific inquiry instead of hanging out at pubs.[165] Likewise, we don't have to let time run through our fingers. How many of our demands could be reduced if we put some energy into prioritizing, organizing, and streamlining the routines that now fritter away our time and misdirect our attention? We can learn to husband time carefully.

Buddhists advise to "act always as if the future of the universe depended on what you did, while laughing at yourself for thinking that whatever you do makes any difference." This serious playfulness makes it possible to be both engaged and carefree at the same time; we can focus consciously on the tasks of everyday life in the knowledge that when we act in the fullness of the experience, we are also building a bridge to the future.

Unfortunately, losing the ability to conduct one's life independently is often a tragic consequence of chronic illness. Yet, even under these circumstances a sense of personal freedom and joy can often be restored. Like a partially polished diamond, some of our qualities, abilities, and virtues are well developed and highly reflective of light, while others remain carbon-coated and dark. Illness is often the catalyst that reveals and shapes the rest of the diamond. A woman in one of our groups had lived a long and rich life in the service of others. As her treatments progressed, she found it increasingly difficult to accept the help being offered. Realizing that her attitude was impacting her joy, she determined to view the undeveloped area of her diamond as an opportunity to experience "the ministry of being ministered to." With practice, she became a gracious and joyful receiver of many acts of loving-kindness. One wise teacher said that psychological health was not to be found in the successful adjustment to one's circumstances, but in the transcendence of them.

Uncovering Hidden Beliefs

Blockages to flow and resonance are often hidden in the form of belief systems from our family of origin. A woman's daughter asked, "Mom, why do you always cut the leg off the turkey and throw it away before you put the turkey in the oven?" "Well, I never really thought about it; my mother always did it. Let's call her up and find out why." The older woman replied, "I don't know why you're doing it, but I did it because I didn't have a pan big enough."

Whether spoken or unspoken, belief systems affect our behavior in powerful ways. Not all belief systems have negative consequences but they frequently operate underground and need to be brought into the light so we can determine if they are still viable and beneficial. At one time, a belief might have fulfilled a purpose but has since outlived its usefulness. For example, some of us might never have learned to read or write or do household tasks if a caring parent had not stipulated that we weren't allowed to play outside until our homework and all our chores were done. While such a rule is effective and even essential for children, as adults the "chores" are never really finished, and that outmoded belief can rob us of spontaneity and pleasure, dictating a life that's all work and no play.

While unexamined belief systems can block feelings of peace and joy or diminish our drive for positive experiences, they can also prove costly in more direct and dangerous ways, blinding us to life-saving action. An hour before sunrise, at 6:01 a.m, on February 9, 1971, while most people slept peacefully in their beds—houses, buildings, freeway overpasses, and hospitals collapsed or caught fire in what would become the third worst earthquake in California history, the San Fernando quake. Lives lost or torn apart by the tremors, smoke, fire, and falling debris would become statistics in the type of earthquake that is most easily prevented: a surface rupture. According to the experts a surface rupture can simply be avoided by not building across active faults. As a result of the extraordinary damage a Fault Zoning Act was created.[166] Now, before a building permit can be issued, a geological investigation must demonstrate that the building will not be constructed across active faults.

Outdated belief systems are like faults in the earth's crust; we need to know where they lie so we won't build on them. The beliefs we hold about our environment and ourselves provide the highest leverage point for our therapeutic interventions because what we *believe* to be true, more than any evidence otherwise, guides our actions and ultimately, the outcome. (Believing that you deserve to live and believing that your body and your medical team have the power to enable you to get well may actually enhance the speed and potency of the healing response.) Unspoken messages from our family of origin, and even our genetic predisposition, influence the frame of reference from which we operate. Unwittingly, just like the woman with the turkey, we can find ourselves stuck in a frame of reference that no longer suits our circumstances or us. These beliefs, especially when they remain unconscious, exert a powerful influence on our behavior, our expectations, and our willingness to embrace a healthier, happier way of being. Uncovering our belief systems is the first step in protecting ourselves from building a future on shaky messages from the past.

Get Started Now: Faulty Belief Systems

Below are a few examples of belief systems patients have shared with me over the years. See if there are any you can relate to, and if so, whether you can determine their origin in your family. Add any others that you may be aware of. Extrapolate and think of the potential consequences of each:

It is selfish to take care of myself.

If you are not going to do it right, don't do it at all.

That's not fair! (Life should be fair.)

Work is work, who says you should enjoy it?

Life is serious business. I must earn the right to have fun.

You cannot play until all the chores are done.

Too many things have gone right lately. Soon, the other shoe will fall.

You can't have everything.

Do not be too happy—something bad will happen.

My doctor is taking care of me; he knows just what to do.

I can't change the past, so why talk about it?

What happens in this family stays in this family.

Hard work never hurt anyone!

Life's a vale of tears.

Some of these beliefs are subtle yet have profound implications. One way to determine what beliefs may be hindering you is to note what behaviors you have difficulty changing (you'll be able to see your reasons for getting stuck). Also pay close attention to when you get upset. An outdated belief system is often behind feelings of disappointment and irritation. Begin with simple areas of life. A pattern of speech or something that routinely upsets you may be a clue to an unproductive belief system. I was called on one of these by my clinical supervisor at Getting Well when someone brought up "life should be fair" and everyone looked at me. "I don't believe that!" I countered defensively. Everyone laughed and I had to listen while various disasters and unfortunate situations were recalled, all followed by my indignant, "Well, that's just not fair." "Oh come on people! I don't *really* believe ..." I sort of trailed off as I got the point. Once we can identify our beliefs we can determine if it is helpful, productive, or congruent with the way we want to live. Then we can choose whether to change the belief or hold on to it.

Affirmations are positive self-statements designed specifically to overcome any negative conditioning from outdated belief systems. They work because we believe what we hear most often about ourselves. One very bright man has dyslexia along with another less common type of learning disability. Growing up, he repeatedly heard, "You're stupid!" If people believed he was brilliant, he thought he had them fooled. No matter how much he achieved, the lingering sense was that his success was accidental. To counter this habitual negativity he chose a reconditioning statement: "I am bright and capable." Generally, an affirmation like this would be said about a hundred times a day for maximum effect. Not to worry—it's easier than it sounds. You don't have to count—just a few times in the shower, on the way to work and the way home and you're done. People report progress after just a few weeks. Writing down your affirmations helps, too. As a rule though, don't work with more than three at a time and make sure that your phrase is stated in the positive all the way around. For example, "I am no longer sick" presents an image of sickness to the picture-making part of your brain. Not something you want! On the other hand, "I feel healthy and full of energy; my body heals and regenerates rapidly" conveys a very different image. Integrating your words with your images gives you an optimal result.

I love the way this poem by Robert Bly wildly illustrates the choices we may not yet recognize and cracks open doors we may have unwittingly closed:

THINGS TO THINK

Think in ways you've never thought before.
If the phone rings, think of it as carrying a message
Larger than anything you've ever heard,
Vaster than a hundred lines of Yeats.
Think that someone may bring a bear to your door,
Maybe wounded and deranged; or think that a moose
Has risen out of the lake, and he's carrying on his antlers
A child of your own whom you've never seen.
When someone knocks on the door, think that he's about
To give you something large: tell you you're forgiven,
Or that it's not necessary to work all the time, or that it's
Been decided that if you lie down no one will die.

—Robert Bly

Symptoms as Metaphors

A shortcut to resonance and interpersonal harmony is portraying a physical symptom as a metaphor, or symbol for any unmet needs. Since the sensitive world of cellular function can mirror the interior landscape of our thoughts and beliefs, our physical symptoms can serve as metaphors for what is happening in our lives. It's not that we cause the problem—that's a popular pitfall discussed in chapter 2. We're not responsible for the symptoms, but we want to be responsive to them so we can upgrade the quality of our life wherever possible.

Family physician Sonia Rapaport routinely incorporates metaphor in her practice. When a group of young girls ran across a freshly paved road, only one developed blisters from the hot tar. While treating her wounds, Dr. Rapaport discovered the girl was about to take her first cross country flight alone to visit her father—standing on her own two feet so to speak. Looking for the metaphor doesn't preclude treatment, but can increase awareness of our part in the healing process. Using my diagnosis of systemic lupus erythematosus (a widespread autoimmune collagen disease), I asked, "In what ways am I attacking myself? What am I rejecting about myself?" This line of questioning continued in my journal until I wrote, "an overactive immune system is like my overactive life." I was so concerned with missing out on something that I routinely overcompensated by doing too much, too often. There are no universal rules here; you are the expert. A client with another type of autoimmune disorder likened it to poor boundaries and not feeling safe to relax. A woman with breast cancer in the left breast associated it with heartache after losing her husband, while another woman connected it with having her children grow up and leave home. Still another related it to lack of nurturing herself. (Not that it has to be related to nurturing at all!) The idea of allergies as metaphor caught one woman's imagination and she began asking herself in what ways she might be "overreacting to life." In the case of asthma a man asked, "Who's taking all my

air?" (In that particular case his adult children were constantly asking
for material and financial help.) One physician encouraged his osteoporosis patients to be aware of any subtle ways they might be devaluing
themselves. Surgeon Bernie Siegel suggests using quiet or relaxation
time to reflect on why the illness is here and what it might be asking of
you.

Our bodies' responses—be they tense breathing, clenched teeth,
stomach queasiness, a fast heart rate, eye twitching, coughing, or clear-
ing our throats—may be a sign of stress or tension that we can tune
into. Since stress is personal, the way it's expressed in our speech is too.
Think about it: He's a pain in the neck. She's going to give me a heart
attack one of these days. Or, I don't want to hear that! One woman diagnosed with neurological Lyme disease (presumably from a tick bite)
noticed she had been saying, "That just really bugs me." More subtle
is the manner in which we refer to the illness. "*My* lupus won't let me
plan that far in advance;" or "*My* arthritis is really getting in the way
of my tennis game." Don't own the illness—just acknowledge it. Sub-
stitute ownership with, "*The* arthritis has flared up but I'll hopefully
be back on the court soon." Or, "Right now I'm taking care of myself
and making plans based on how I feel in the moment." One woman
said, "I'm a healthy person who happens to be dealing with (fill in the
blank.)" Refine what you say to yourself and how you say it, because
your body is listening.

Other beliefs are not so easy to penetrate. Steve had lost both his
father and grandfather to heart disease at an early age. When Steve was
fifty-two he suffered a massive heart attack that left him literally with
only half a heart. After much reflection, he chose to consciously uncover
and evaluate the beliefs he held about his genetic potential and then actively cultivate faith in his ability to transcend his biological inheritance.
He also closely examined any resistance he experienced while trying to
change his lifestyle. For Steve to change his diet and begin an exercise
program, he had to believe such acts could make a difference in his life

and that it would be worth it. Furthermore, to maintain such discipline he would have to have many things to personally look forward to and be actively engaged with living. Most importantly, he would have to determine if he felt deserving of living a full and productive life.

At eighty-two years of age Steve shared that story with all of us in the program. He did dramatically change his eating habits (he said his rule of thumb was if it tasted good he spit it out!). He walked three miles every day. When he retired he joined a bowling league and traveled often. He refused to accept a prognosis of inactivity and early death and his love of living served as a powerful motivating force for personal change.

Now, a watershed study by the CDC (Centers for Disease Control) brings to light other hidden factors that can undermine your health. Vital to beating the odds, discover how you can protect yourself in the very next chapter.

Week Four

Immune Power: Insight and Your Extraordinary Life— The Writing Cure!

The intuitive mind is a sacred gift and the rational mind is a faithful servant. We have created a society that honors the servant and has forgotten the gift.

—ALBERT EINSTEIN

What began as the trip of a lifetime on an adventure vessel ended in the icy waters of the Antarctic Peninsula. On November 23, 2007, most of the hundred passengers were sleeping soundly when the impact came. The noise was deafening as the *MS Explorer* rammed into a chunk of ice and water began pouring in. Panicked and freezing, passengers were packed into lifeboats and four frigid hours later were rescued by a Norwegian cruise ship.[167]

For ships in these waters it's not the gigantic drifting bergs of ice that pose the greatest danger, but the smaller chunks of ice that are nearly undetectable to radar. In fact, only 10 percent of the mass of an iceberg is above the surface of the water. What is seen can be circumvented. However, like the unseen portion of icebergs below the ocean's surface that sink great ships, our childhood experiences can impact our adult health in monumental ways.

How We Know: The ACE Study

A landmark study, the largest of its kind linking stress in early life with disease in adulthood, was conceived, not in the hallowed halls of a fabled university, but literally on the backs of paper napkins during dinner.[168] The story begins in 1975 when Dr. Vincent Felitti founded the Department of Preventive Medicine at Kaiser Permanente in San Diego, California. Overseeing fifty-eight thousand people a year for comprehensive medical evaluations, Dr. Felitti realized that certain problems did not fit into the conventional medical model and other interventions were needed. And so in 1983, along with a pharmaceutical company, he developed a nutrient-based fasting program for the treatment of obesity using the supplement Optifast™. Individuals lost record amounts of weight—up to an astonishing three hundred pounds per year without surgery—but a surprising number of the successful fled the program. Dr. Felitti described to me how the counter-intuitive dropout rate left researchers astonished and scratching their heads.

Not having a sure trajectory as to where this was going, Felitti started interviewing people in depth, asking all manner of questions including, almost as an afterthought, how old they were when they first became sexually active. The first person he asked began sobbing, telling him she only weighed forty pounds when she was sexually molested by her father. Ten days later when another patient reported incest, he decided to routinely inquire about sexual abuse. Later, after dozens and dozens of similar accounts, he became convinced of the relationship between morbid obesity and deeply wounding childhood experiences. One hundred and eighty-six patients later, he had a solid 55 percent link between major obesity and childhood sexual abuse. Ruling out bias, five other interviewers came up with the same statistic in an additional one hundred patients.

In 1990, Felitti had an opportunity to present his findings at a conference in Atlanta, Georgia, and was "wildly attacked by the audience," which interestingly enough, was comprised of many psychologists who believed the tales of abuse "were just cover stories for failed lives." Later that evening, Dr. Felitti found himself seated at dinner next to David Williamson, Ph.D., of the CDC (Centers for Disease Control). "David said to me, 'This is a provocative study and of enormous importance for the country as well as the practice of medicine, but no one will believe you based on a limited sample of two hundred and eighty-six people, no matter how well you have studied them. We need thousands of people from a general population.' So we decided, then and there, on the back of a paper napkin, what history and which labs and what physical evidence we would need, and designed a second questionnaire relating to adverse childhood experiences."

Who Gets Sick

In this updated version of a comprehensive medical history, the focus of research was no longer obesity, but matching the current health of the patient with any reported adverse childhood experiences. Incidence of heart disease, cancer, or other chronic illness, along with lifestyle factors such as promiscuity and street drug use were all integrated. While Kaiser's existing built-in tracking mechanism and health care plans meant researchers didn't face an insurmountable financial hurdle, they did face a significant challenge getting the study approved through the Institutional Review Board (IRB). The IRB critiques nearly all the studies that you read or hear about and is designed to protect the rights and well-being of test subjects. In this case the IRB responded, "You can't ask people questions like that—it will cause them to decompensate." So

Dr. Felitti and his team responded by offering to provide 24-hour phone support to all participants. The IRB agreed and the ACE (Adverse Childhood Experiences) Study was approved.[169]

Ten categories of adverse experiences in childhood were selected, based on their prevalence in the weight program. One unexpected revelation was how many patients in a general, middle-class population were raped, molested as children, or had someone in their family who was murdered or in prison. Then there were issues of neglect—there might be someone who would feed, buy clothes for, and send their child to school, but the child's clothes would be dirty and he might not be taken to the doctor when he was sick. Or there was domestic violence. So ultimately the study tracked these and other types of emotional and physical neglect or abuse along with traits of dysfunctional households.

As the results began streaming in, Dr. Felitti said, "The magnitude of the relationships surprised even me—the increased incidence of disease was often in the hundreds of percents and occasionally thousands of percents. The epidemiologists of the CDC said those were the magnitudes that would occur once in a lifetime for an epidemiologist." Epidemiology is a highly regarded cornerstone of public health, the specialized study of illness across the population. Robert Anda, M.D., M.S., came to the CDC as an epidemiologist in the 1980s just as it was building its capacity to thoroughly investigate chronic illness—the biggest killer in this country—not just infectious disease. When the opportunity came to analyze Felitti's initial findings Dr. Anda confided that he was skeptical but intrigued, and so he spent six months researching abstracts of child abuse and neglect. "The literature was fragmented—bits and pieces not pulled together. I could see that we needed a broad based public health study including as many health issues as we could measure." He was willing to risk being fired to work on the project because of "… the potential it held and my sense that the conceptual framework for the leading causes of death was changing right before my eyes." He was right.

While the published research includes more than seventeen thousand participants, Felitti tells me that, "To date, over the past eight years, four hundred and forty thousand patients have completed our new medical questionnaire that incorporates questions from the ACE Study. The children who were traumatized or suffered neglect or abuse while growing up were over one and a half times as likely as others to develop heart disease, coronary artery disease, or cancer in adulthood."

Anda explained that the risk factors for the leading causes of disease are not randomly distributed. It's not a roll of the dice, but a rigged game that has more to do with childhood experience than anyone could have predicted. The numbers turned out to be huge. In this relatively well-educated upper middle class population two-thirds had at least one ACE (Adverse Childhood Experience). More than one in ten had five or more ACEs. The cumulative impact is in the statistics: as the ACE score increases so does the risk of numerous health problems. For example, a higher score on the ACE questionnaire more than doubles the risk for ischemic heart disease (reduced blood supply to the heart) above and beyond all other traditional risk factors such as cholesterol or smoking. The percentage keeps rising in perfect step with the elevated ACEs.

This vital information clearly hasn't trickled down yet to mainstream sources. By way of example, chronic lung disease (Chronic Obstructive Pulmonary Disease or COPD) is projected to be the third leading cause of death worldwide. But if you look up chronic lung disease or ischemic heart disease on Wikipedia, ACEs aren't even mentioned—yet the risk for COPD is two and a half times greater with an ACE score of four versus an ACE score of zero! But what about traditional risk factors like smoking? With an elevated ACE score there is a 200 percent increase *not* accounted for by smoking, and with heart disease an increase was seen in the hundreds of percents, unrelated to cholesterol or obesity! The increase in these big killers (as we've seen before in other studies) was independent of all other risk factors including obesity, smoking history, high blood pressure, and high cholesterol. While autoimmune diseases are less common in the population, the research is "strongly suggestive" of a link with the ACE score. Dr. Anda continues, "I was blown away." They were looking at a national health issue.

Healing the Past in the Present

But what about the clinicians who were on call 24/7 for the respondents in the study—how many phone calls did they receive from people who were decompensating as a result of answering a questionnaire about their childhood experiences? "Not a one. Not one single phone call. I do have, however," Dr. Felitti continued, "a notebook of letters, mostly thank you letters, from elderly women who wrote to me saying, 'Thank you for asking. I feared I would die and no one would know what had happened to me.'"

While the impact of the study lies in its size and the strength of its findings, the beauty of it lies in its totally unexpected clinical significance. A company on the New York Stock Exchange specializing in neural net analysis, and trying to move into the medical field offered, as a gift, two years of follow-up on one hundred and twenty thousand participants who had undergone a comprehensive medical evaluation using the new ACE-based questionnaire. I felt a chill run up my spine as Dr. Felitti laid the results before me: There was a 35 percent drop in doctor's office visits, an 11 percent drop in emergency room visits, and a 3 percent drop in hospitalizations compared to the year before. What did they believe accounted for the result? Dr. Felitti replied, "That's hard to answer definitely. But I can tell you what all of us associated with this work believe. We were asking, and people were telling us the worst secrets of their lives, and they were still accepted as human beings." Despite the astounding results, a peculiar difficulty arose. Newspapers and some media were reluctant to publish the questionnaire for fear of upsetting people. The participants responded themselves and below is an amalgam of just two of the many letters Dr. Felitti received:

I have read the questionnaire over and over. I have been thinking a lot about it. I had a difficult childhood very similar to what Christina Crawford described in her book *Mommie Dearest*. I feel that if I had this questionnaire in front of me years ago I would have come forward to get help and would not have blamed myself for every bad situation that happened to me. As it was I suffered for years. I hope that you do publish the questionnaire because I know that you would help a lot of hurting people that otherwise would never talk about their difficult childhood. The mind is very powerful. I was told every day that I was worthless and would never accomplish anything in life. If the questionnaire had been put in front of me it would have shown me that the people in the medical profession knew about the sad things that happen to some people. I am fifty-three years old now and it has only been about ten years ago that I started allowing myself to think that it was OK for me to enjoy life. I am seeing a psychologist, taking antidepressants and have joined a theatre group. I still have a long way to go, but I can see a big difference in my life. I am setting boundaries and standing up for my rights. How many [more] lives can be saved by this program [questionnaire]?

You can take the same questionnaire these participants did at this CDC site: www.cdc.gov/nccdphp/ACE/

Children who grow up in spring-loaded environments, where their need for vigilance remains fairly constant, have a higher rate of illness over all. As it turns out, a particular genetic marker involved in serotonin function (5-HTTLPR) is associated with added vulnerability to trauma when two of its components (alleles) are short in length. Presenting a very specialized view of the matter is Yale Professor of Psychiatry Joan Kaufman, who found that the genetic vulnerability was expressed *only* in the children who were maltreated.[170] Going back to what we learned about gene expression, we can see that environment can trigger a genetic consequence as well as lend a hand in making amends, for in those genetically vulnerable children, a supportive male influence proved helpful in recovering emotionally.

More evidence was revealed in 2008 when a possible link between child abuse and asthma was found. In a collaborative study between Brigham and Women's Hospital in Boston, the University of Puerto Rico and specialists from Columbia University, researchers discovered that children who are abused physically or sexually are twice as likely to develop asthma as those who are not mistreated.[171] In a tragic legacy, abused children are more likely to grow up to maltreat their own children. Reversing that trend, Dr. Anda is bringing this information into the school system so parents can take the test themselves and better protect the health and well-being of the next generation.

For our purposes, the tantalizing implication is that we're only as healthy as the secrets we share. This, in and of itself, isn't necessarily new information. Twenty years ago investigations revealed that upheavals "kept secret were more likely to result in health problems than those that could be spoken about more openly."[172] What is new, are the variety of immune markers and physical health measures that track positive changes following an emotional disclosure and are likewise associated with significant drops in physician visits. Science writer Henry Dreher captures the power of disclosure under the subheading "Truth or Dare: The Health Effects of Opening Up" in his book *Mind-Body Unity*.[173] A leading expert on the physical effects of confession, James Pennebaker, Ph.D., professor of psychiatry at the University of Texas, interviewed polygraph instructors and learned "…of a peculiar but telling sequence of events that typically occurred when individuals guilty of a crime were given a polygraph test. When people are initially hooked up…whether guilty or not—their autonomic nervous systems are racing, with elevated heart rate, breathing rate, blood pressure, and skin conductance. …When a confession is induced…in most instances he or she is required to take one more polygraphs to ensure that the confession was truthful, and it is here that the peculiarity occurs. Although at that very moment the person's life is in a shambles, remarkably he or she is often found to be physiologically very relaxed. The person's heart rate has slowed, breathing has slowed, skin conductance has normalized, and blood pressure has lowered. Often the suspect warmly thanks the polygraph instructor before he or she is carted off to jail."[174]

The Yellow Brick Road

When healing, our task isn't to carry the past as a torch, but to integrate it into our consciousness so we can mend the trauma and move forward. Sharing our story can be part of the healing. I witnessed this first hand when I attended Harvard's clinical training program in mind-body medicine. It was reported that victims of trauma had lower levels of physiological arousal after spending a few consecutive days repeating their story. After telling the details over and over, to person after person, in a compressed period of time, the trauma appears to lose some of its punch. As attendees, we tried this ourselves, and took turns speaking about the most traumatic memory we had, to one person at a time, sharing and listening, then moving on to the next person in the group. The older gentleman before me was strong and self-assured, a physician specializing in integrative medicine, but his voice quivered when he told me that when he was eleven-years-old he was attacked on the way home from school by a stranger and left for dead under a pile of leaves. He had disobeyed his parents and taken a short cut through the woods where a man beat him into unconsciousness, and believing him to be dead, covered his body in a shallow grave. Regaining consciousness a few hours later, he told his parents he was targeted by bullies at school rather than risk their displeasure at his disobedience. After retelling the story over and over again, he found that what began as a difficult emotional task became a transformative one, as the rote recitation changed his relationship to the actual experience into an almost casual one. "After back-to-back recounting, the story took on a tedious quality and I found myself rushing through the narrative. ...'and then I was covered with leaves and left for dead'...as if it wasn't so much about me but about a past that no longer pushed my buttons in quite the same way." (See the Resource Guide for more on trauma.)

While there is no one-size-fits-all solution as the ACE and Spiegel (chapter 2) studies remind us, the tremendous value of disclosure cannot be ignored. In the experiment above, instructions were clear for the listening mode: only empathetic, supportive statements, no advice-giving or personal anecdotes, just being present with tender attention. This is another possible explanation for the healing effects—the unconditional acceptance of those we share with. And it may not be our friends or our family who can provide this (they may not be able to stop themselves from advice giving or judgment), but we may find unconditional acceptance in the healing ear of a kindly physician or nurse, a stranger, or the supportive arm of a group, bound together not by blood or by beliefs, but by stories of adversity and triumph. In the story telling we weave together disparate and broken parts of ourselves into a courageous tapestry of grace and meaning, and in doing so, come to honor who we are because of where we've been. Until now, traditional training for physicians has focused primarily on symptoms rather than stories, but at Columbia University's College of Physicians and Surgeons, Rita Charon, M.D., Ph.D., chairs a program in "Narrative Medicine," showcasing the importance of story-telling when healing.

The specific method of sharing may not matter much. In an unusual project, seventy-two rheumatoid arthritis patients were split into two groups. One disclosed their deepest feelings about something stressful and the second group spoke about their thoughts of neutral pictures. Both groups spoke into a tape recorder for fifteen minutes a day for four consecutive days. Three months later when evaluated at a clinic, the group that disclosed their emotions functioned better physically in daily life than did the control group. But in a surprising twist, those who reported negative feelings or emotional distress *after* doing the task had the greatest joint improvement of all.[175] Although the process was painful, long-term improvement was documented. While we can only speculate as to why that's so, a participant in one of the six-week classes offered, "We can only heal what we can feel."

Writing for Your Life

Talking isn't the only coin-of-the realm when it comes to the healing properties of disclosure.[176] The literature is packed with evidence that suggests you can write your way to better health. So compelling is the data that in 2002 the American Psychological Association published a book summarizing the findings titled *The Writing Cure.*[177] Abundant evidence demonstrates that expressive writing (or journaling) boosts thinking ability; increases working memory; reduces pain, tension, and fatigue; enhances mood and sleep quality; and positively influences your immune system. Best of all, it's free and requires no special skills, and you can shred whatever you write and still get all the benefits.

Consider a study with patients suffering from asthma and rheumatoid arthritis who either wrote about the most stressful event of their lives or neutral topics, for just three sessions. Physical evaluations performed four months later showed significant improvements in lung function and joint mobility for those who wrote about emotional events but no real improvement in the control group.[178] Likewise, in a study of healthy college students, those who kept journals of feelings instead of just activity diaries had more active immune systems for up to six months after journaling stopped. This may be because expressive writing techniques can assist in resolving inner conflict that can sabotage the inner peace and tranquility necessary for deep healing. In one study, college students were asked to write about a personal trauma while another group of students wrote fictional accounts of trauma. In the following month, researchers found that the students who wrote about personal traumas made two-thirds fewer trips to the doctor than did those that had written the fictionalized accounts.[179]

Our more immediate response to distressing memories or thoughts ("unpleasantness" as some of my southern friends say) may be to sweep them under the rug, out of sight, out of mind, distracting and distancing ourselves from the source of our discomfort with Moon Pies or heaping portions of banana pudding. (As a Midwestern friend said, "Only in the South; we just aren't that into bananas here.") While that sort of distraction may work for us in the short term, it can have poor long-term consequences as unhealthy behaviors of all kinds rise with avoidance. A growing body of evidence indicates that while a stiff upper lip and stoicism may be valued in our culture, repression can carry quite a high price tag. In a study of more than one thousand people over a forty year period, researchers at John Hopkins University in Baltimore discovered that students who had a "limited expression of tension or anxiety" were twice as likely to die by age fifty-five as their peers who were either able to express anxiety or experienced little tension![180] No one is advocating that we exploit nervous tension, but there are serious medical advantages to identifying our feelings, and then dealing with them.

By avoiding upsetting information we unwittingly set ourselves up for more difficulties later. Over time, suppressing unwanted thoughts and feelings can consume our physical and mental resources, so there's less to go around for problem solving and creative thinking. Not surprisingly then, research reveals that expressive writing improves working memory, a term used to describe our ability to stay focused and on task. Multiple studies clearly indicate that writing about negative or traumatic events is more effective in improving working memory than trivial writing.[181] We can only guess at the mechanism, but it may be that sitting on top of smoldering emotions swallows up precious energy resources that become available once we recognize and resolve inner conflict.

To appreciate how this might work, imagine that you are sitting in one of our group classes and on your way home have to stop by the grocery store for several items you need to pick up. If you recall, it's the job of your subconscious to alert you to unfinished business, so from time to time during the class you are prompted to remember this or that at the store. But what if you had a list of all the items you needed to pick up? Just knowing that these things are written down allows your mind to relax and focus on the present. In a similar fashion, journaling, even about things beyond our control, gives our subconscious the message that it is taken care of and it becomes easier for us to move on and let go. What though, as if flying beneath the radar, our emotions are undetected, operating outside of our awareness?

Unlocking the Truth

In 2007 if you Googled the Chinese translation for *flippant*, you would get, "The assassin who stabbed Bush." According to *New Scientist* magazine the error likely resulted from a defective algorithm.[182] Computer programmers build algorithms (rules or processes) into their software to produce accurate calculations. But a breakdown in the logic or the formula can result in some pretty wild feedback. In this case, if you couldn't speak English you wouldn't know there was a problem and you would literally be lost in translation, all due to a funky algorithm. Likewise, if we are unable to accurately label what we feel, it might be time to adjust our algorithm or we too can get lost in translation. The good news is that if we aren't well versed in the language of feelings, we can learn. At least one study shows that exercises that help us identify feelings can even reduce our risk of cardiac problems.[183] By developing this awareness, a whole new world opens up before us. When Helen Keller was eighteen months old, scarlet fever left her blind and deaf. She was seven before Anne Sullivan began working with her. In her own words Helen describes her first grasp of language:

Miss Sullivan had tried to impress it upon me that "m-u-g" is mug and that "w-a-t-e-r" is water, but I persisted in confounding the two...We walked down the path to the well-house...and my teacher placed my hand under the spout. As the cool stream gushed over one hand she spelled into the other the word water, first slowly, then rapidly. I stood still, my whole attention fixed upon the motions of her fingers. Suddenly I felt a misty consciousness...and somehow the mystery of language was revealed to me. I knew then that "w-a-t-e-r" meant the wonderful cool something that was flowing over my hand. That living word awakened my soul, gave it light, hope, joy, set it free! ...Everything had a name, and each name gave birth to a new thought. As we returned to the house every object which I touched seemed to quiver with life.[184]

Like learning a new language, some feelings can be so disguised or buried that we have to look for physical clues. Unconsciously denying negative feelings results in physiological arousal that can be measured by biofeedback, EMG, EEG, temperature, and moisture.[185] You may not consciously feel disturbed by low levels of depression or anxiety, but your cold hands, back pain, or headache may signal otherwise. Getting curious about your physical symptoms can open the door to identifying and exploring emotions—which can lead to releasing and resolving them.

When one man began to keep a journal for the first time, a certain pattern of behavior revealed itself. Every Friday night he picked a fight with his wife. Once the pattern became part of his awareness, he was able to relate the outbursts to the turmoil he experienced as a child when he had to leave his father's home and spend the weekend with his mother, with whom he had a troubled relationship. Your journal can help you identify the psychological events (stresses, interactions with people, etc.) that influence both your mood and your body. Writing down what symptoms you experience, and when you have them, helps connect the dots. Then, once a week you can look back on what you've written and notice any connections between events, moods, and symptoms. (Of course, you need freedom from prying eyes. For writing to be truly therapeutic, it must be free from censure.)

If emotions are kept from conscious awareness, can they affect our DNA? Possibly. The choices we make and the interpretation we assign events can influence physiological outcomes. Awareness opens a window for new perceptions, and subsequently, new molecules of emotion to circulate with potentially different results. But what if your feelings are hard to define? Initially it may help to break down feelings of vague discomfort into one of four main categories of unpleasant feelings: anger, sadness, fear, or hurt. Then search for a word on the feelings vocabulary list (in the Resource Guide) that most accurately captures the nuance of your feeling. Consciously create an environment of non-judgmental awareness around your discoveries. Feelings just are; they're not right or wrong, they just exist. Acknowledging our feelings—not indulging them—gives us the clarity and insight to transform any latent negativity or unfinished business into an opportunity for personal growth and healing. The silver lining in a painful process is expressed by a participant in the six-week class who wrote to me, "When I journal frequently, I can quickly figure out why I have 'that feeling' in the pit of my stomach. I may be angry, or someone has said something that hurt my feelings, but I haven't thought about it consciously—I just have 'that feeling.'"

The Heroic Journey

Lisa's medical history was not long, but it was complicated. Pain, blurry vision, brain fog, and an intractable, weighty fatigue, exacerbated by the inability to sleep, sent her to two infectious disease specialists before she was diagnosed with chronic fatigue syndrome. With treatment she felt a measure of relief, but her cortisol (an adrenal stress hormone) levels were abnormal, so her physician referred her to me. We began with diaphragmatic breathing, and each week or so we would add another tool or strategy to her cache of self-healing skills.

As Lisa became relaxed, she began to open up about her childhood. Her father wasn't at home during her growing up years; as a result, her mother had raised Lisa. Rather than being sent to her room or going without dessert, Lisa was hit with belts, paddles, hair brushes, and yard sticks regularly over a period of many years, until she was fourteen or fifteen years old. Like many who were brought up in stressful environments, Lisa's childhood memory is riddled with holes. And if it weren't for the kindness of the community, Lisa might never have found validation for the memories she has. After Lisa became seriously ill, a few people came forward and shared with her what they had witnessed (violating the boundaries of other families, Lisa's mother had even spanked and disciplined other women's children in public).

In high school, a kind teacher took a close personal interest in Lisa and allowed her to accompany her on museum visits, theater trips, and outdoor adventures, all rich and varied experiences that she appreciates to this day. But one night, while she was asleep on the teacher's downstairs sofa, the woman's husband raped Lisa. Drenched in shame, she shouldered this unspoken burden for decades. During that time, the years seemed to roll one over the other, moving from grace to trauma and back again. Lisa and I added other supports and she also saw a clinical psychologist for some testing. (In the Get Started Now exercise, "Three Steps for Moving On," you can read about one of the tools Lisa used.) When we concluded our work together, Lisa was having longer periods free of pain and fatigue and was reconnecting with former interests and hobbies. It was some time before I heard from her again. One day when opening the mail, I found an invitation to her first gallery exhibition. Since then, she's had several showings and her work is carried in at least two galleries. When we spoke, Lisa said, "My program of self-care is my priority because it allows me to be the person I was always meant to become."

Get Started Now: Three Steps for Moving On (Adapted from Interapy: A Model of Therapeutic Writing Through the Internet)[186]

As with all exercises and suggestions, write only what you feel safe in disclosing.

Step 1. Write quickly and with abandon (ignoring spelling, grammar, etc.) as you describe in detail the problem, disturbing event, or trauma. Uncensored, allow yourself to write anything you like to the person or people involved. Don't hold back, this isn't a letter you'll send! When you've completed that, engage in something relaxing or distracting, a walk or a hot bath, or read something uplifting. If possible, the next day move on to…

Step 2. If your dearest friend or child had suffered the same, what would you want them to know? What advice would you have for them? What might they have learned from the event? Have they grown in any way or was there a benefit to the crisis? What might your friend have learned about himself or herself from going through this difficulty? Pretend you are responding to your friend or child and write out your words of hope, comfort and advice. The next day move on to…

Step 3. Symbolically take your leave of the past and move forward by composing a letter to yourself or to someone involved in the distressing event. Rewrite as necessary, so that the finished product is so immaculate and dignified that you could potentially mail it if you chose. It's not necessary to read or send the letter. You can burn it—symbolically releasing all that it represents—or bury it, or seal it away in a private place.

One man felt it important to read his letter to his parents, and they both apologized. "We could have done so many things better," they said. Those kind, compassionate, and humble words helped heal the emotional rift that had developed over the years. On the other hand, when Lisa wanted to read her letter to her mother, she was cautioned by her psychologist to scrutinize her motives. He warned her that if she was going to do this, it needed to be for Lisa alone, not in a hopeful expectation of receiving an apology or hearing an admission of guilt. As you might imagine, Lisa's mother reacted with indignation and justified her behavior. Lisa moved to plan B, and you already know the ending.

Dysfunctional households are often characterized by severe boundary violations—putting children at an increased risk of illness in adult life. Dr. Felitti (of the ACE Study) stressed that there was a "strong graded relationship" between dysfunction in the family and the child's health in adulthood. Like others, Atlanta psychologist Dr. Roger Buddington uses a standardized test, originally designed by the military—the Minnesota Multiphasic Personality Inventory (MMPI)—when beginning counseling with a new client. While the MMPI can detect psychological disorders, it can also pick up on trauma—not the type of trauma, but the intensity and prolonged exposure to stressors that can sometimes result in posttraumatic stress disorder (PTSD) in children and frequently remain hidden as they grow up to become seemingly high functioning adults. Although Lisa minimized the rape (since she was seventeen when it happened, she thought she should just "get over it") and her childhood spankings (she said, "it's not like I was locked in a closet"), Lisa's MMPI was no different than someone who had been ritually sexually abused. Trauma can be just that, regardless of the source—encoded in the psyche and measured by a standardized test.

Get Started Now: The Five-Day Advantage

Researchers at Harvard Medical School found significant mental and physical health benefits in cancer patients who wrote their deepest feelings and thoughts for thirty minutes every day. Positive results were seen after only four consecutive days of writing.[187] For optimal benefit, you need to feel free from censure, so find a quiet and secluded spot and write with abandon—avoid playing hide and seek with how you really feel. Write freely, without worrying about spelling, grammar, or sentence structure. Unlined drawing pads make great journals so feelings can be expressed through squiggles, scribbles, and drawings. If you have a distressing topic in mind, you'll naturally know when you're ready to move on because the item will lose steam, and one day, maybe tomorrow, maybe next week, you won't be writing about that issue anymore.

If there's nothing in particular you'd like to write about, try a technique called stream-of-consciousness. Writing faster than you can think, the idea is to keep your pen moving even if what you write makes little sense (you may doodle or scribble, but keep your pen moving). In this technique, whatever pops into your mind finds a place on the page until you feel a shift and begin writing about something that may have needed expressing. Your writing may look like this: "My coffee's getting cold; look at the laundry piling up over there; I need to bathe the dog; I had an interesting dream last night..." It doesn't really matter. In this valuable technique, what needs to come out usually does. There's no need to keep what you've written or reread it. You can shred it or throw it away, especially if you're concerned about prying eyes. Write for five consecutive days and then evaluate your experience. The most important thing is to do it. (One caveat, this kind of writing can be stimulating and isn't the best before bedtime. If you want to write before bed, a list of what you're grateful for will put you in a fine frame of mind for refreshing sleep.)

A good friend of mine prefers to do her journaling at the zoo. She has a tendency to save up six months worth of material for a frenzied one-day journaling extravaganza surrounded by animals behind bars. She usually chooses a day during the week when the zoo will be quiet, so she can hear herself think. The last time she went it was so cold and rainy the gorillas wouldn't even come out (but they were smarter than the orangutans; she sent me photos of one standing wet and miserable out in the rain with his poor little hands over his head). This must have given her some serious food for thought because she didn't stop journaling even when the zoo closed. Walking to a Chinese restaurant she ordered a martini (in a Chinese restaurant?). Three employees frowned over the recipe book as they tried to concoct a Cosmo. Yet she kept writing. I'm not suggesting that you give yourself tendonitis by writing all day in the damp, cold weather (yes, she had tendonitis for at least a week) and my friend says it doesn't have to be the zoo—but she recommends "an enjoyable place where you can relax, calm down, and let the thoughts flow with ease."

A steady stream of ideas, stories and inspiration come out of our ongoing group meetings at the cancer center. Graduates of the six-week program can meet monthly if they choose, and I adore the energy, stimulating discussions, debates, and hearty laughter we share. And despite moans, heavy sighing, and eye rolls, we occasionally engage in journaling or another expressive therapy exercise together. Some of us have been meeting regularly now for more than a decade. Marquita Foster is one. An artist and inspirational group member, she has spearheaded some of our most interesting projects. Bringing in boxes of feathers, sequins, shells, buttons, and bows along with markers, paint, and glue guns, she handed each of us a muslin doll. For about fifteen or twenty minutes we pinned, taped, and glued all manner of accoutrements on our doll and then passed it down to the person next to us. Each doll had a wristband with a tag, where each of us working on that doll would contribute to the storyline. With shells for shoes, wings, and feather headdresses—some anatomically correct, and others hoping to be— they are a magnificent collection. Clipping a hook to each doll and hanging them on a decorative rod, we created the most spectacular sight in our group room. So when Marquita sent me the following excerpt from *The Blackberry Tea Club* by Barbara Herrick, I took notice: "Six days of journaling won't do it, but six months out you begin to notice that you are different, and people respond to you differently. In six years, nothing in your life will be the same. You'll explode miserable relationships and nightmarish jobs, and pick your way through the debris, word by tenuous word, until you find a better place to plant your feet, like mountaintops and long straight roads to the horizon."[188]

You may surprise yourself with what you can do with journaling. When faced with the challenges of healing, we need creative problem-solving abilities as never before. The very same tools and techniques that writers, artists, and playwrights use can strengthen our problem-solving skills and heighten intuitive awareness.

Give Yourself a Breakthrough

One simple technique called clustering is found in many course books on writing, as it is a brainstorming technique (Gabriele Rico, who authored *Writing the Natural Way*, coined this phrase[189]). Starting with one word, write as many words as you can think of that are associated with the first word. It does not matter whether or not they make sense. The key is to keep your pen moving. Soon, you will feel a shift and get a sense of what you wish to write about. When that happens, just let the words flow. In this week of the program the word we happened to be clustering was *marriage*. The words a patient wrote were: *house, children, share, love, peace, happiness,* and *health.* Then the words that followed were: *dominating, orders, humiliation, embarrassment, criticism,* and *no attention.* Then she quickly wrote the following vignette:

Marriage as I See It

Marriage as I would want it, would be to share a life with someone you love and have a house and children, all living in love with peace, health and happiness, communication, understanding, and compassion...and lots and lots of hugs. Marriage should not be a one-way street with a dominating figure as a father barking orders and humiliating and embarrassing and criticizing me. And giving no attention to me as if I was not even there. Used as housecleaner and call girl and secretary and nurse maid and taxi driver, cook and servant.

The spontaneous nature of expressive therapy (art, movement or writing) often sparks something that might not come up in a traditional talk therapy session. Once a submerged issue comes to light, it can be processed and resolved. Self-limiting beliefs can be exposed so we can operate in our best interest. Uncovering what may be missing in our lives can prompt us to identify and meet our own needs and goals. In the process, writing, art, and imagery can overlap and poetically merge. For example, when clustering, a group member shared this:

> I was like a song with unfinished lyrics,
> The music could have been sweet and heard
> Far and wide if I had allowed it to be sung.
> The lyrics could have told of strengths and beauty
> And love from within but they were not yet written.
> The tune could have been like that of the song of
> A bird but I hadn't learned yet to fly high enough and was
> Afraid to be heard.
> Now I sing aloud and I will be heard.
> I will be cherished.

Expressive writing, drawing, and other techniques help us to, as Anne Sexton said, "Put your ear down close and listen to your soul hard." Doing so, we begin to feel more connected to ourselves, accepting our past and embracing our future. To illustrate the cumulative value, I asked a group of patients to write a list of words that would describe themselves. (Why not try this now?) One man wrote:

> smart, thoughtful, analytical, pleasant

For the next week everyone in the group practiced imagery, journaling, and some other type of expressive therapy such as painting or drawing. On the seventh day, I asked the group members to write another list of words that described themselves. This time, the same man's list was:

smart, great sense of humor, lovable, pliable, flexible, normal, moral, hopeful, wishful, thorough, bright, colorful, thoughtful, noisy, witty, keen, analytical, creative, intelligent, playful, pink, cute, motherly, fatherly, skillful, talented, devoted, self-taught, learning, caring, squeezable, helpful, capable, story teller, ill, truthful, looking for love, looking for approval, a thinker

The list grew from four adjectives to nearly forty in just one week! The corpus callosum connects the right and left hemispheres of our brain, sponsoring a free flow of information and consequently, creative leaps of intuitive awareness and problem solving. A sense of exhilaration often accompanies these flashes of insight. The upshot is greater self-awareness and the ability to see connections between things that were previously viewed as unrelated. Imagery, deep relaxation, and expressive writing or drawing can give you a leading edge in your quest to beat the odds.

A Happy Medium

As you can see, all this writing isn't just about bad news. Some research indicates that dwelling on emotion alone can be counterproductive in terms of health.[190] The findings, though, aren't necessarily counterintuitive to what you've just been reading. For journaling to be truly therapeutic, more than venting is required. The key lies in exploring the relationship between the experience (the event itself) and our feelings about it. It makes good sense if you think about it. While focusing exclusively on what's wrong in our lives can lead to feelings of depression, ignoring the same can make us vulnerable to nasty surprises. In fact, it's easier to find and preserve the good when we've had plenty of opportunity to acknowledge, address, and process the disappointments. Dealing with what is—even if it's unpleasant—and then moving on to appreciate and express gratitude for all the good things in life keeps us moving forward in a positive direction. Shedding light on our past can lead to reframing the trauma, even constructing a new "ending" to the story we've created in our mind.

Writing about how you've changed or grown as a result of your experience has its own cache of benefits. A few years ago, ninety-two women who had completed treatment for breast cancer were followed for three months. Investigators found that forming a cohesive story of a traumatic event in writing resulted in less disability from illness. Those who shared and wrote about the meaning they found in the experience, along with its trials and stressors, had fewer medical appointments, a stronger self-image, enhanced vigor, and less emotional distress than the less expressive women.[191]

Bearing this out is a five-year follow-up study of women with breast cancer conducted by researchers at the University of Miami. In their analysis, women who managed to find some benefit in the experience reported less depression and a better quality of life overall when compared to those who could find nothing positive.[192] Some of the benefits were discovering who their dependable friends were, becoming a stronger person, and discerning a larger purpose in life. Further research reveals that writing about your "best possible self" resulted in a significant boost in mood for participants along with a drop in illness when compared to those who wrote about neutral topics.[193] Yet not all studies support a positive outcome from benefit finding. If participants were suppressing painful emotions, this could, in part, explain the result. For these reasons, it's prudent to try a variety of techniques and always trust your own sense of what is appropriate for you.

On the other hand, without any apparent contradictions, several studies indicate that keeping a gratitude journal can be good medicine, positively affecting us mentally and physically, resulting in symptom reduction and fewer medical visits.[194] When facing any level of loss, it can be extremely rewarding to focus on all that might be right with us—

no matter how small—and on the blessings we do enjoy. One woman keeps a beautiful, leather bound gratitude journal on her bedside table and every night before going to sleep she records all the sweet moments, the great and the small pleasures of her day. Since doing so, she finds herself not only noticing such times but actively searching for them, knowing they will all be captured at the end of the day in her special book. Now this is a journal you don't have to shred! (For another, see the Get Started Now exercise "The Best Year of Your Life".)

Get Started Now: Boost Your Mood

When you feel discouraged, any one of the journaling exercises below can help you turn the page. Choose one and notice how you feel. For a serious boost, try one each day for three consecutive days.

1. Give yourself permission to close your eyes and take three deep, cleansing breaths. Visit your healing place and allow yourself to get comfortable. When it seems right to you, imagine how you would like to see yourself in the future. What sort of life dreams would you like to see fulfilled? What is your philosophy of life? What do you see happening? Imagine that all of these dreams came true and that everything working out well for you. How does it feel? Is there anything you would like to change? Now write about your experience, fleshing out your dreams for the future with as much detail as you can.

2. Describe your most meaningful experience—and why.

3. Write about something that went well in the last week. Who was ultimately responsible for that goodness? (Nine times out of ten, it's you!)

Sweet Dreams

We've all had dreams about nerve-wracking experiences—cramming for an exam, speaking in public, or running from danger. And whether you're going through an emotional divorce or have just returned from the frontlines, your dreams can reflect your hopes, your fears, or the nightmare of battle. After a shocking diagnosis or a traumatic surgical procedure, disturbing dreams can rob us of a peaceful night's sleep just when we need it the most. For optimum health, a certain amount of time each night needs to be spent in rapid eye movement or REM, the state in which our most vivid dreams are recalled. Unfortunately, the benefit can be lost if our sleep is plagued by intensely disturbing dreams. (As an aside, recent studies show that children and teenagers who do not get adequate amounts of sleep miss out on valuable REM and as a result have a significant increase in obesity.)[195]

Not surprisingly, brain imaging (scans) during periods of dreaming show intense activity in the area of the limbic system, the area that helps regulate moods and feelings.[196] Cancer specialist Mitchell Gaynor, M.D., the director of medical oncology and director of integrative medicine at the Strang Program for Cancer Prevention and an assistant clinical professor of medicine at the Cornell Medical Center in New York, encourages patients to record their dreams. Repetitive or recurring dreams can zero in on an area of conflict and furnish a shortcut to a constructive solution.

A friend of mine was an attorney in San Francisco when he had a recurring nightmare. Either locked in a jail cell or sentenced to prison, he was trapped behind steel bars with no way out. He wrote me, "Besides jail, sometimes I was on the run from people trying to imprison me, other times I was semi-free but in a tyrannical country in which I was fleeing. But always trapped or fleeing entrapment." Once he left the legal profession to pursue an alternative career, the dream vanished. I've experienced this myself. When I lived in New England, circumstances required that I relocate every year or two. When it came close to moving time, my sleep was peppered with repetitive dreams about not being able to find my shoes, or all my stockings were torn, or I could find one shoe but not its mate. After talking about these dreams with my clinical supervisor, I started doing some imagery with my feet "planted firmly on the ground," along with some supportive affirmations. The dreams came to an end, and I felt more confident about my upcoming move. In these instances, the dreams become a springboard to examine life issues that may need our attention so we can raise questions, forge a new path, or simply gain a fresh perspective.

When diagnosed with ocular melanoma (a deadly cancer of the eye), internationally recognized scientist and imagery pioneer Dr. Jeanne Achterberg left no stone unturned as she searched for metaphor and insight in expressive writing, recurring dreams, and imagery. There were no easy answers, but she couldn't ignore the fact that she was rapidly losing her eyesight, and as a psychology professor and senior editor of a national journal, she spent a great deal of time critiquing the work of doctoral students and reviewing submissions—taxing her already overburdened vision and further draining her physically. Other epiphanies followed, building over time until the sum total of her quest led to leaving Santa Fe altogether and accepting a research position at a hospital in Hawaii. Today she's healthy, renewed, and recharged for a brand new life.

While professional help is recommended if you're suffering from PTSD (posttraumatic stress disorder), the book *Crisis Dreaming*, by Rosalind Cartwright, Ph.D., and Lynne Lamberg, recommends this natural tool to restore peaceful sleep and gain more control in our emotional lives when we are facing a crisis—divorce, sickness, financial problems, or other distressing challenges.[197] The key is simple: Just fix any dream that is upsetting by creating a new ending. Even if the dream is over and you are wide awake, make up an ending that's personally empowering for you. (For me, in addition to an appropriate affirmation, when I woke up I fixed my recurring dream above by imagining that I had matching shoes that fit and my stockings were all perfect.) At the very least, choosing a more suitable ending to your dream leaves you feeling better for the rest of the day.

From these examples, you can see the real meaning behind any dream is in the eye of the dreamer. In a journal article, Barbara Dossey, Ph.D., a pioneer in the field of holistic nursing, related the story of a man who shared his dream featuring a skull and crossbones just two nights before he was scheduled for open-heart surgery.[198] She asked him to tell her what he thought it meant. As it turned out, he was worried about what would happen to his wife if he died—he didn't have a will, his wife knew nothing about his investments, and she didn't know how to write checks. Barbara pointed out that it was unlikely that he would die during the surgery, especially if he prepared by eliminating anxiety and fear. She helped him find a lawyer to take care of the essentials and encouraged him to tell his wife about the investments. Notice that Dr. Dossey did not offer a personal interpretation or assign meaning to symbols, but simply asked the man what the dream meant to him. You are always the expert on your symbols!

Get Started Now: The Best Year of Your Life

One of my best buddies happens to be young, happy, and in great health. But she doesn't take it for granted. Despite her good fortune, she realizes that life can be fragile and unpredictable, so she has an ongoing wish list that contains her near and long-term dreams—things she wants to do before she "kicks the bucket." Another friend and I get to go along for the ride, so to speak, on her adventures. From having high tea at the Ritz-Carlton to hiking up Stone Mountain in the dark to watch the sunrise, we adore taking part in her list. With that spirit in mind, put aside all your to-do lists and clear a space that allows you to focus unencumbered for a moment. Imagine that this is the last year of your life. With paper and pen, write what you would like to experience this year. What would your year consist of? Initially write with abandon, as if you were brainstorming and no idea is excluded, no matter how farfetched. Then look over what you've written. Assuming that you can't just quit your job or move to Tahiti, what realistically could you do this year? It may mean more picnics, an adventure trip, or spending time with old friends. Create a fresh list of goals. Put it in your calendar or planner and work what you can into your life. It just may be that, by doing this, every year is your best year yet. If you enjoy these exercises, the books listed in the Resource Guide will provide you with more ways of exploring and mining the gifts of your creative self.

Drawing Upon Your Experience

Developing our creative potential isn't as complicated as it may seem and can be pleasurable. Three techniques—music, imagery, and expressive therapy (which includes writing, drawing, and Marquita's muslin dolls!)—all have a cumulative and positive effect. When transforming a health issue, drawing may offer additional advantages. David was only twenty-seven years old when he was told that his cancer treatment had not been effective and he had less than three months to live. At Getting Well he expressed the loss and sense of utter hopelessness by drawing himself as a dying rosebush with all the petals scattered on the ground and the specter of a tombstone behind it. Later, as he began to experiment with some of the methods you've been reading about, he drew himself as a multicolored, eight-foot torch of life with a constantly burning fire. He saw this as his indomitable spirit and his will to live. David didn't die as predicted. I had the privilege of meeting him a few years after his astonishing recovery, when he was collecting stories and interviewing other people who beat the odds.

Our drawings are not prognostications, but tools for personal discovery. Like expressive writing, where we're not concerned with grammar or punctuation, the more childlike are our drawings, the more potent and effective they can be. In working with professional artists, I always encourage them to draw spontaneously, even using their non-dominant hand for a while. Then, look for the metaphor in the drawing and ask yourself a few questions about what you notice. If the hands are missing in a drawing of yourself, don't blame it on not being able to draw hands, but ask different questions such as, "Since the diagnosis, how am

I meeting my own needs?" Or if the dark cloud is right over your head, "What in my life feels like a looming storm?"

A young woman with two small children had a rare type of lymphoma and had been undergoing chemotherapy off and on for over three years. She drew herself riding her bicycle, but those of us in the class noticed that she had drawn herself as if she were invisible. The group members asked her if she noticed that the bicycle was visible through her skin and clothing. She hadn't thought about it, but reflecting more deeply, she said she couldn't see her future, and therefore could not make any plans. The group then asked how she would act and feel if she knew she had longer to live. At that moment, she realized that she'd been missing out on the present—not allowing herself to savor the moment or celebrate the fact that she was still alive. She died several years later, but not before teaching us that *living with* is different from *dying from*.

Two drawings that were on the wall of our group room speak for themselves. When asked to draw a picture of himself healthy, one group member drew a picture of a bodybuilder, similar to Atlas, with the world on his shoulders. Another drew a picture of a man, hands on hips, head looking down, in a contemplative manner, but standing on the world. One has the weight of the world on his shoulders, and one is on top of the world. This provoked a lively discussion in the group about responsibility and how we choose to shoulder it.

Some folks get a little nervous about what may be revealed in their drawings. But as with icebergs, knowing where trouble may lie gives you the control and the power. Looking at what is, you can accept it, process it, or change it. For maximum insight, I've found it helpful to put my drawing away for a week or two and then bring it out again, maybe putting it up on the refrigerator or the bulletin board in my office for a fresh look. More often than not, I notice something completely new and different than I did the first time around.

Other people, though, aren't limited by my point of view and can immediately give me an original take on what I've drawn—this also keeps my perspective from getting stale. In one exercise, I worked along with everyone else as we drew totem poles with the faces we present to the world and the ones we conceal. When we were finished someone asked me, "What in your life is like a fish bowl?" At the time I was going through a very public divorce, and sure enough, each of the faces I drew looked like they were in a fish bowl!

Get Started Now: Act as If

Psychoneuroimmunologist Nicholas Hall uses the following exercise to show how the combination of acting skills, imagery, and music can change our physiology. Begin by rating how you feel now on a scale of one to ten. One is the worst feeling possible, and ten is a fabulous feeling. Now play a piece of music that is sad, and imagine the saddest moment of your life. Imagine where you were, what was happening, how you looked, and how you carried your body. Immerse yourself in the feeling of sadness. After one minute, rate the sad feeling on the same scale of intensity. Now do the same process for the opposite emotion. Imagine that you have just won a championship or the sweepstakes, or that you have accomplished something grand against insurmountable odds. Play a piece of music that echoes your feeling of triumph. Rearrange the muscles in your face. Assume the posture that would accompany such a remarkable moment. Absorb that feeling of victory. After one minute, rate this new feeling. What we imagine, how we act, and the music we listen to all exert a powerful influence on our mood and orientation toward life, as well as on our immune system.

Unconscious conflict or physical signs can be a clarion call for expressive therapy techniques. After incorporating one or more of these methods into their routine, people report new insights and speedy problem-solving, and a greater connection to the here-and-now; and all the colors, sights, and sounds around them seem more vivid. As an added bonus, art-based activities can bring about a euphoric effect that can last for hours. Whether you're healing the past in the present, facing a turning point in the here-and-now, or carving out a new vista for the future, expressive techniques can clear your vision, open your heart, and leave you feeling gloriously unencumbered. Opening the door to insight can be fun, exhilarating, challenging, even intimidating at times, but always offers an opportunity for embracing the extraordinary in the life you're living now.

The broad scope of healing interventions you've read about so far can all change our internal milieu, lower stress hormones, and help regulate the autonomic nervous system. Coming up, you'll discover traits that counteract the sense of vigilance and heightened arousal of early childhood conditioning and take advantage of a simple technique that can remap connections in the brain, creating new opportunities for healing and learning. But in the meantime, the very next chapter takes you into the heart of survivor research, where simple strategies yield powerful results.

Week Five

8

Survivor Traits: What They Are, What They Do, and How to Get Them

It is much more important to know what sort of patient has the disease than what sort of disease the patient has.
—SIR WILLIAM OSLER (FATHER OF MODERN MEDICINE)

The young boy was suffering from a usually fatal blood disease, requiring long hospital stays and sometimes-painful procedures. But one evening when the nurse came to take his vital signs she found him sitting on the floor with a surgical mask on. He resisted her best efforts to get him back in bed:

> "I'm dying anyway. …Ever since I got in that bed, I've been getting sicker. I'm not going to stay in it any more." "Come on, be a good boy. Get back in bed and take off that mask." "No way!" shot back the boy. "The doctors wear these things to keep the sickness out of them and they never seem to get sick at all. From now on I wear this all the time. Just call me the masked patient. Who is that masked boy?"…[Dr. Pearsall continues:] On rounds the next day I found Danny huddled inside an elaborate tent. His bed had been stripped

bare to the mattress, and on a bedpan hung from the IV rack was a sign which read, "No germs or night nurses allowed." ..."Can I talk with you, Danny?" I asked.

"If you come into my secret healing place," he answered... "This is my healing place. I feel safe; I think I can get better here. My parents can come in, and you can come in, and Jeff the cleaning man can come in, but that's all." "Can Dr. Caster come in," I asked. I knew that special dispensation would be required to enter this newly erected temple. "Only if he knows my new password," was Danny's response. When I asked for the password, Danny slowly lowered his mask, leaned forward, placed his arm around my neck, and muttered into my ear the magical word to enter his new world. Over the next two weeks, with continual grumbling by the hospital staff, from dietary services to respiratory therapy, Danny conducted his hospital business from his healing place. He exited only for tests with those who knew the password... [And at the end of two weeks] his blood disease had gone into remission.[199]

Would you like to know what his password was? It was his name, Danny. Taking charge of a tragic situation can harness the healing power of the human spirit in marvelous and mysterious ways. Danny defied protocol. Despite judgment and persuasion he defined the parameters of his healing environment and ultimately took control of both his life and his immune system. Control is a key component of certain characteristics known as "survivor traits." These attributes are linked to an extraordinary ability to ward off illness, even in the face of extreme duress.

How We Know: The Science of Survivorship

Going beyond mere concept, the data is rich—compelling us to look closely at the damaging effects of helplessness and hopelessness and the pivotal role of control in beating the odds.[200] A young graduate student in the late 1970s set the pace with what would become a landmark study. Madelon Visintainer took three groups of rats and implanted each with a certain number of cancerous cells, so that under normal laboratory conditions it could be predicted that 50 percent of the rats would go on to develop a tumor and 50 percent would be able to throw it off. In this experiment, one group of rats received mild shocks that they weren't able to escape or do anything about; the second group received the same sort of shock but were able to learn to avoid it, while the third had no shock at all. As expected, within a month, half of the rats in regular, laboratory rat life had a tumor and half were healthy; of the rats that had uncontrollable shocks, over 70 percent developed a tumor; but remarkably, of the rats that were able to master the shock by pressing a lever to avoid it—only 30 percent succumbed.[201] This is stunning. The immune systems of rats that had control were more vital and responsive than rats that received no shock at all. As you'll see, it is not the events of our lives that have such weighty impact on our immunity, but our feeling of mastery over them.

Even more impressive are studies with people where large survival benefits are linked with small changes in daily life. In one such study, nursing home residents were either assigned to care for a plant of their choosing or had their plant maintained by the staff. In just a few weeks a measurable upturn was documented in the folks taking personal responsibility for their plant. More astonishing though, a year and a half later only 15 percent of the plant caring group had died—compared to 30 percent of the other![202]

Leading up to this juncture were two psychiatrists in the 1960s, Thomas Holmes and Richard Rahe of the University of Washington Medical School, who were anxious to know whether there was a connection between life events and future health. After examining five thousand medical charts, they culled a list of events that had occurred prior to the onset of illness. Death of a spouse, losing one's job, relocation, marriage, the birth of a child—forty-three life events both heartening and harrowing were tallied. Through statistical analysis, based on the health of the patients, a numerical value was assigned to each event. The number of points accumulated during a twelve-month period predicted who would be most likely to get sick—the higher the score, the greater likelihood of illness. The test, called The Life Events Checklist (LEC), and its predictive accuracy became well known, popping up in *Readers Digest* articles and cementing the relationship between stress and illness.

But what about the people who, despite great stress and high numbers on the scale, didn't get sick? Curious, researchers turned their attention to how they might be different. Clinical psychologist Suzanne Kobasa and her colleagues at City University of New York discovered that these individuals exhibit a strong "commitment to self, an attitude of vigorousness toward the environment, a sense of personal meaningfulness and a feeling of being in control of their lives."[203] She labeled these men and women "stress-hardy" and defined three distinct traits that were common among them and designated them the "three Cs" for Control, Commitment, and Challenge. The exciting news is that the characteristics of stress-hardy folks like Danny can be learned or adopted by less stress-hardy folks like, well, me for instance. The three Cs can be used in different ways and circumstances to boost your own level of stress hardiness.

The concept, though, is not without conflict. The authors of a leading ten-year study on coping style and cancer write, "The possibility that psychological response … can influence the outcome of the disease is a contentious issue." Yet they forged ahead evaluating "helplessness/hopelessness, fighting spirit and depression" in early-stage breast cancer patients. Ten years later it was found that neither depression nor the holy grail of cancer jargon, fighting spirit, had any significant effect on survival—but feelings of helplessness and hopelessness did—and negatively so.[204] Helplessness cripples our capacity for self-protection, rendering us vulnerable to the vagaries of circumstance and paralyzing our ability to respond. Overall results demonstrate that people who stay healthy sense that they can influence what is going on in their lives—at least to a degree—like Danny. Gaining a sense of control is easier than you might think. In fact, you've already begun.

The Three Cs

If you are following the six-week program, over the past few weeks you've catalogued new areas of control: raising your hand temperature, adjusting an attitude, releasing the past, and choosing beliefs that are in your best interest, to name a few. But taking control isn't solely about our inner world. Even from the crucible of a cancer ward, by establishing control Danny created a cascade of corrective internal chemicals. In part this was accomplished by altering his backdrop for getting well—his hospital bed.

When researching this aspect of the three Cs, I quickly discovered a wealth of data about the impact of our surroundings. A well-designed study recently reported in the journal *Neuron* showed that subconscious messages (which we pick up on from our environment) influence decision-making.[205] Take a close look at your own healing domain, whatever it may be—a house, a room, or a flat. Imagine that you're looking around with the detached eye of an observer and notice what sort of messages you've been sending yourself. We may not consciously think of the particular experience or story behind each item in our home, but the subliminal message of every color, piece of furniture, or art is registered and recorded. For example, if you or a friend has had chemotherapy, then you only have to think of that particular shade of yellow (the color of the i.v. therapy) to know that our environment exerts an effect on our emotions. Cancer centers are advised not to paint their walls the color known as "chemo yellow." (And for good reason!)

The effects of subliminal messages can be profound. In a Harvard research project elderly people were exposed to fleeting messages linking positive qualities such as wisdom and experience to the aging process. With what result? After a short time they began walking with increased stamina and vigor. The measurable improvement was so great it matched the results that would be obtained in a twelve-week exercise program![206]

So take a careful inventory of the messages contained in your environment. Is the story behind the object one you want to be reminded of? Photographs, art work, and gifts, like music, can operate in the background and keep you rooted in the past or moving forward toward the future. One woman always felt sad in a particular room. Upon closer reflection she realized most of the contents were the hard-won spoils of a contentious divorce. Molecular biologist Bruce Lipton, an international authority in cellular communication at University of Wisconsin School of Medicine, doesn't think we should take our surroundings lightly. In his workshops he emphasizes that if we make personal changes but our environment doesn't change along with us, we are energetically pulled back to where we started.

Experiment with your surroundings. Notice how you feel in particular spaces outside of your home and incorporate any positive aspects you find into your plans. De-clutter, maximize flow, and prioritize. Whether it's a poem on your refrigerator or a flower in a vase, make sure the message you're receiving is an encouraging one. In a recent investigation, researchers at Texas State University conducted a survey of more than four hundred office workers and found that those who kept at least one plant in their office were happier and more satisfied with life in general than those without a plant.[207] Whether it's a room or a healing corner, the color, art, and message should inspire and refresh. When I needed most to believe in what appeared to be an unlikely recovery, I kept this poem where I could see it daily:

This is about power. The tremendous power of lightning and thunder. The power of an ocean wave crashing on the shore. The power of a million suns blazing in the sky. The amazing power of the human mind and body to regenerate. The power of nature. The power of understanding, compassion and love.

—Albert Marchetti, M.D.[208]

Curiosity, Novelty, and Enrichment

Another way we take control of our environment is through enrichment. That can mean anything from a change of pace—an outing, a vacation, or altering your daily routine—to learning a foreign language. Visiting an art or science museum, going to the opera, seeing a play, or taking a walk through a nature center are all activities that refresh and revitalize your worldview. But more than that is at stake. Psychobiologist Ernest Rossi explains that novelty and enrichment stimulate growth of nervous tissue in the brain and facilitate genetic (genomic) expression.[209] So any opportunity for enrichment can ultimately be a healing one. If there's something you have always wanted to learn about, now may be a good time to rekindle your curiosity. (It's easier than ever now that many universities offer free access to certain online courses.)

The three Cs can be adapted to almost any circumstance. Last summer, in a freak medical accident, I lost two thirds of my blood through a hemolytic process. Put simply, my body was destroying red blood cells faster than I could make them and in less than one week I had lost nearly all of my blood. In the emergency that followed, I learned something about helplessness. The specialists told me that under optimal conditions I would make enough blood to be back on my feet in four or five weeks. Until then, I had so little blood volume, walking more than a few feet could result in cardiac failure.

It was under these circumstances that my husband and my friends went to the library and the bookstore. I had the books, journals, and magazines they brought me on the floor, the bedside table, and in the bed. There were books on communist China (something I knew nothing about), a biography of George Eliot (never had a chance to read about her), and some overly ambitious material on quantum physics that confused me. A good friend added a few mystery novels for entertainment and some Sudoku puzzles to keep the frustration level up and I was good to go. Reframing my confinement as an opportunity to learn, I was excited to wake up in the morning—first, because I woke up at all, and second, because of all the engaging things I was reading about. (With nowhere to go, I finally got around to loading my CD library into my computer, and it's worth mentioning that I was also on heavy-duty steroids, so was pretty hyper if you hadn't already guessed.) I like to believe my enthusiasm paid off; four weeks later I was back at work and the next week hiking in the North Georgia mountains.

Whatever the level of loss, a chronic illness can provide a unique vantage point to prioritize your life. Speaking at a function, I noticed a tiny woman a few rows from the front nodding her head vigorously as I spoke. Intrigued, I interrupted myself and asked if she would be willing to share what was on her mind. She had been diagnosed with widespread cancer, and despite chemotherapy and radiation, things stayed about the same. Anxious and depressed, she kept asking her doctor, "Please, tell me—how long do I have?" "He never would tell me, but one day he just sat me down and said, 'Let me give you a piece of advice—you just go ahead with living—live your life. Do whatever it is you've always wanted to do.' I decided then and there that I'd take his advice. That was eight years ago and I've been doing just that ever since."

Which Brings Us to...Commitment

The second 'C' in the three Cs is Commitment: Commitment to yourself and what you are engaged in. Like Control, we manifest Commitment to ourselves in many different ways. One of the most compelling examples comes from Dr. Seth Yellin, chief of facial plastic surgery at Emory Healthcare in Atlanta. Yellin is passionate about trusting a patient's instinct about their own well-being—encouraging patients to tell him how they really feel. It's a position born of experience. When the tables were turned and he knew he needed medical treatment, he was hassled—and then ignored.

When Yellin was chief resident in head and neck surgery at Cornell Medical Center he woke up early one morning and while shaving, felt a mass in his thyroid gland. He kissed his wife who was still in bed and said, "I have thyroid cancer," and then went on to work. There he endured the special cynicism reserved for young doctors who become convinced that they have whatever disorder they happen to be specializing in. Yet Yellin insisted on a thyroid needle biopsy. More heckling arose when the results came back non-diagnostic—not negative and not positive—and he was encouraged to simply take a watch-and-wait approach. Convinced otherwise, he insisted upon an ultrasound guided needle biopsy and, when no one would order it, he ordered it himself. But again, the finding was non-diagnostic. Ironically, during a free moment between thyroid surgical cases that he was performing on others with cancer, Yellin went to the pathology lab and examined the biopsy slides himself. He immediately recognized that there should be more tissue slides than what he was seeing. Sure enough, two slides were missing. After locating the slides, which had been misfiled, the pathologist—right then and there—diagnosed him with thyroid cancer. Yellin knew his body, trusted his instincts, and didn't rely on the approval of other people or wait for someone to agree with him; he took control, exhibited a high level of commitment to himself, and acted as if he really mattered.

Years later, these same instincts would save the life of his young son. It was a brisk winter day and Dr. Yellin was dressing his two-year-old son for a quick trip to get bagels for brunch. Slipping the toddler's baseball cap on, he noticed that it fit snuggly, more so than just a few weeks before. Later, when his son complained of a headache and pointed to the right side of his head, Yellin didn't waste any time. During the evaluation that followed, the pediatric neurologist measured the child's head and acknowledged that while it was a bit larger than average, it was nothing to be concerned about and recommended reevaluating him in another six months. Trusting his own intuitive awareness, Yellin insisted on further diagnostics and on January 19, 1999, a brain tumor was discovered, compressing the ventricles and causing increased pressure on the brain. Nine years and many surgeries later, his son, "a miracle child," is doing well in school, athletically, and socially, and recently played the piano and sang at the Brain Tumor Foundation for Children's fundraiser.

You don't have to naturally be a Danny or Dr. Yellin. Early research seemed to indicate you were either a survivor or you were not. We now know that these traits can be learned and the effect is the same as if you had been this way from the day you were born. Like other skills, you can learn to trust and believe in yourself and remain committed to what you know to be true. This chapter introduces you to survivor traits that can be learned, adopted, polished up, or even pulled out just when you need them most and with the same net gains as if you came by these traits genetically.

In fact, just acting as if you matter can provide a powerful cue. The simple trick of adjusting your facial expression has been shown to correspond with changes in both your mood and in your blood serum. Backing this up, when actors were assigned by researchers to play various roles, their blood chemistry levels reflected the particular state they were acting out. And when they acted happy, certain immune cells were enhanced.[210] In another project researchers demonstrated that deliberately choosing a particular facial expression had a marked effect on the autonomic nervous system, which controls breathing, heartbeat, and digestion.[211] No one's recommending suppressing your emotions—we've already discussed how damaging that can be. But once we've acknowledged what we feel, we can adopt a particular attitude to help us meet our goals. Don't let the simplicity fool you—it's a powerful technique—and can be useful in a variety of situations.

Recently, when asked to read an excerpt from this chapter to a small group of friendly people, I was startled at my trembling hands and shaking voice. Later, when I calmed down I realized that when I speak to a group, it's usually a fluid experience, with a lot of give and take. I can back up and use a new illustration if my point isn't clear. Better yet, I can quote someone else. Reading words that I've written didn't allow for going back or re-explaining or quoting someone fancy. What I would be reading were my words, fixed in black and white, and they would have to stand all on their own. Identifying the source of my self-doubt didn't help. In a few days I needed to be able to read an excerpt to a larger audience. There wasn't time for a deep analysis; I needed a quick fix and "acting as if" was it. I decided that author Kathleen Brehony would be my role model of choice. Confident but not cocky, I've seen her poised before groups both large and small, and fast enough on her feet to do a bit of standup comedy when the situation demanded it. And she reads her words with confidence and poise. "Acting as if" I was Kathleen Brehony, the evening reading went off without a hitch (no Valium required).

This simple strategy can help us develop both Control and Commitment. You can get a sense of this now by choosing an emotion you would like to display. Is there someone that can inspire you? Adjust your posture, your breathing, and your facial expression accordingly and notice how you feel. (We'll take a deeper look at the third C, Challenge, in the next chapter.)

Survivor Traits

Psychologist Al Siebert has made a career of studying the characteristics of all manner of survivors, from prisoners-of-war to individuals triumphing over a catastrophic diagnosis. His interest began in 1953 when he joined the paratroopers, where the characteristics of survivors surprised him:

I was sent to Ft. Campbell, Kentucky, and assigned to the 503rd Airborne Infantry Regiment for basic training. As part of the 11th Airborne Division, the 503rd had returned from Korea after suffering heavy losses in combat. We were told that only one in ten men had come back alive. These were jungle fighters—tough, unstoppable, and deadly. They would be our training cadre, and we were nervous about what our training would be like. Talk of mean, screaming drill sergeants spread through the barracks.

When we started basic training, however, the sergeants and officers were not what we had expected. They were tough but showed patience. They pushed us hard but were tolerant. When a trainee made a mistake, they were more likely to laugh and be amused than to be angry.

Combat survivors, it turns out, are more like Alan Alda playing Hawkeye, the mischievous, non-conforming surgeon in the M.A.S.H. television series, than they are like the movie character Rambo. The commanding officer of SEALS training at the Naval Special Warfare Center, for example, said in a magazine interview, "The Rambo-types are the first to go."[212]

After his infantry experience, Dr. Siebert interviewed hundreds of people: survivors of death marches and the Nazi Holocaust; ex-prisoners-of-war and Vietnam veterans; survivors of cancer, polio, head injury, and other physically challenging conditions; survivors of abuse and alcoholism; parents of murdered children; as well as survivors of bankruptcy, job loss, and other major life-disrupting events. What he learned was that most survivors are ordinary people, who faced extraordinary situations and rebuilt their lives by tapping into their deepest strengths and abilities. Another distinguished survivor researcher, psychologist Julius Segal, said, "In a remarkable number of cases, those who have suffered and prevail find that after their ordeal they begin to operate at a higher level than ever before. ...Those terrible experiences of our lives, despite the pain they bring, may become our redemption."[213]

Dr. Siebert has generously allowed us to reproduce his Resiliency Quiz for you to take.

Get Started Now: How Resilient Are You?

Developed by Al Siebert, PhD.

Rate yourself from 1 to 5 on the following: (1 = very little, 5 = very strong)

___ In a crisis or chaotic situation, I calm myself and focus on taking useful actions.

___ I'm usually optimistic. I see difficulties as temporary and expect to overcome them.

___ I can tolerate high levels of ambiguity and uncertainty about situations.

___ I adapt quickly to new developments. I'm good at bouncing back from difficulties.

___ I'm playful. I find the humor in rough situations, and can laugh at myself.

___ I'm able to recover emotionally from losses and setbacks. I have friends I can talk with. I can express my feelings to others and ask for help. Feelings of anger, loss, and discouragement don't last long.

___ I feel self-confident, appreciate myself, and have a healthy concept of who I am.

___ I'm curious. I ask questions. I want to know how things work. I like to try new ways of doing things.

___ I learn valuable lessons from my experiences and from the experiences of others.

___ I'm good at solving problems. I can use analytical logic, be creative, or use practical common sense.

___ I'm good at making things work well. I'm often asked to lead groups and projects.

___ I'm very flexible. I feel comfortable with my paradoxical complexity. I'm optimistic and pessimistic, trusting and cautious, unselfish and selfish, and so forth.

___ I'm always myself, but I've noticed that I'm different in different situations.

___ I prefer to work without a written job description. I'm more effective when I'm free to do what I think is best in each situation.

___ I "read" people well and trust my intuition.

___ I'm a good listener. I have good empathy skills.

___ I'm non-judgmental about others and adapt to people's different personality styles.

___ I'm very durable. I hold up well during tough times. I have an independent spirit underneath my cooperative way of working with others.

___ I've been made stronger and better by difficult experiences.

___ I've converted misfortune into good luck and found benefits in bad experiences.

_____ Total

Scoring:
80 or higher = Very resilient
65–80 = Better than most
50–65 = Slow but adequate
40–50 = You're struggling
40 and under = Seek help!

For a description of each item in the above questionnaire take a look at Dr. Siebert's website at www.resiliencycenter.com.

From The Resiliency Advantage by Al Siebert, PhD

Reprinted with permission.

Assuming you've taken the quiz, what can you do if you would like your score to be higher? Acting "as if" can help you here. Since feelings often follow thoughts and behaviors, a short-cut to practicing commitment to yourself is to imagine someone else in your shoes. Someone you care deeply about. If your best friend or your daughter were in your situation, how would you want them to consider themselves? Would you want them to push, prod, and berate themselves? Exhaust their mind and body? Deprive themselves of good things? Pause a moment to ponder how you would treat yourself if you really mattered. Then turn that around—and act as if you are that friend or that precious child—and give to yourself the grace and appreciation you so readily give another. Acting as if you matter creates optimal conditions for the authentic feeling to flourish. Learning to take Control and developing Commitment to one's personal well-being are essential ingredients for a lifetime of self-care. In scrupulously examining how she treats herself, one woman with an autoimmune disease said, "I look at the whole month in my planner, checking for balance. Is it too full of commitments? Too much work, study—too much of anything? Do I have enough 'free' Saturdays to do what I feel like doing? Am I getting enough play in my life?" Which brings us to another survivor strategy—having fun.

> *All the days of the afflicted one are bad; but the one that is good at heart has a feast constantly.*
>
> —PROVERBS 15:15, *THE KING JAMES BIBLE*

The Healing Power of Laughter and Play

Being committed to ourselves and engaged with life means packing in plenty of laughter and play. The intricate web of relationships between brain chemicals and virtually all the systems of our body can be seen by tracking the effects of laughter. Humor not only feels good—activating regions of the brain associated with happiness and euphoria—but can give us a valuable edge when beating the odds. Dr. Lee Berk of the Loma Linda University Medical School in California, a pioneer in psychoneuroimmunology, verifies that hearty giggles and belly laughs enhance the immune system, increase natural disease-fighting killer cells, and ward off stress-related illness.[214] It's no wonder that backed by dozens of studies, the American Psychological Association asserts that a healthy dose of humor is good medicine.[215]

Specifically, laughter has been found to activate T-lymphocytes, increase production of gamma interferon (an immunity-strengthening hormone), reduce levels of the stress hormone epinephrine (which in turn, lowers high blood pressure and cortisol), and even help regulate heart rhythm.[216] Bearing this out, a cardiologist at the University of Maryland Medical Center, Dr. Michael Miller, found that people who use humor and laughter regularly are more likely to have healthy hearts than those who don't.[217] In one study, two groups of cardiac patients were followed for a year. While both groups received standard-of-care treatment, the group that watched a funny video for thirty minutes a day had fewer arrhythmias (irregular or abnormal heart rhythms) than the control group.[218] Research shows that the advantage may stem from the way that hearty belly laughing allows blood vessels to expand and contract more effectively. On the other hand, stressful movies appear to have the opposite effect, narrowing and restricting blood flow by as much as 35 percent.[219]

We may not think too much about the function of our blood vessels in our day-to-day lives, but new findings hint of noteworthy discoveries yet ahead. Dr. William Fry, psychiatrist and professor at Stanford University, has studied the effects of laughter for decades. In a recent communication he explained, "Arterial functioning is far more complex than we ever suspected it to be. ...One colleague of mine at Stanford has proposed that arteries should be recognized, as a physical entity, as another endocrine organ, with complex secretory and reactive functions. Very exciting stuff!" Stoking speculation, Drs. Fry and Miller (the cardiologist mentioned in the previous paragraph) will be publishing a paper on their conclusions next year.

More research by Fry places laughter and play firmly in your medicine bag of tricks. Consider, for example, his study where hearty laughter was shown to increase levels of circulating antibodies—an important component of immunity—for up to thirty-six hours.[220] Spotlighting other effects, Fry and colleagues demonstrated that just one minute of mirthful laughter can equal ten minutes on a rowing machine![221] Further findings show laughter may even provide protection against free radicals. Free-radical scavenging capacity, as measured in saliva, rose an average of 30 percent after watching a single episode of a half–hour comedy.[222] And in patients with rheumatoid arthritis, dissolving into hearty laughter rapidly lowered interleukin-6 levels by half (a marker of inflammation), suggesting that this could influence the neuroendocrine-immune system in a positive way.[223]

Humor can also be helpful in dealing with the dark side of things. Listening to the peals of laughter coming from our group room, nurses in the hallway frequently ask what could possibly be so funny in a support group. As with a lot of this kind of humor, you really have to be there. But to give you an idea, Dick Haddow, a Scotsman you'll meet again in the last chapter, said he didn't think he should die before he had worn out all his body parts. Every now and then the group would receive a letter from him (when unable to attend our monthly meetings) signed, "Haven't worn out all the body parts yet!" There was also a crazy, long, curly, red wig that got passed around. It would disappear sometimes for months at a time and when we least expected it, someone would trounce into the room in some unbelievable getup. One woman came in looking as if she were ready to perform at the Grand Ole Opry, and Dick gave us all a start when he walked in as "Dixie." (At 6'4" he was quite a sight since he used chalk as makeup, but he had quite a shock himself when the watercolor paint he used to imitate nail polish wouldn't come off. It had to grow out!).

Dr. Jaime Sanz-Ortiz, a specialist in cancer and palliative medicine, summarizes that while humor strengthens immunity in addition to reducing pain, anxiety, and tension, it also inspires creativity and hope and distracts us from our problems—even if it's only for a moment—and gives a fresh perspective to our concerns (whatever they may be).[224]

So look for ways to cultivate humor, search out wonder, and add more laughter and play to your day. Give yourself a healing edge by taking a break from the newspaper or the evening news. Play a game or just practice laughing. At least for one physician, no jokes are needed. Madan Kataria, M.D., author of *Laugh for No Reason*, finds health advantages just from going through the motions.[225] If you would like to dial up your humor quotient, explore the tapes and videos by Loretta LaRoche, M.D.,—the Mirth Doctor. Her website is listed in the Resource Guide.

Acting as If You're Worth It

When we allow ourselves healing intervals throughout the day—whether through laughter, diaphragmatic breathing, or by taking an imagery break—our body picks up on this subtle energy and gets the message that we matter. Tuning in creates a pause; we can rethink an automatic assumption or reflect on a habitual response that may not be in keeping with our own best interest. Since our bodies require raw materials to make needed repairs, acting as if we really matter means adhering to nutritional guidelines and getting enough exercise (see the Resource Guide for current thinking in these areas). Of course optimal nutrition can't correct the risk factors of helplessness and hopelessness. Likewise, all the mind-body medicine in the world won't protect you from scurvy if you're stuck in the middle of the ocean without any vitamin C.

But information isn't the problem, is it? We usually know what is good for us; it's no great mystery that we should be eating more fruits and vegetables, and rejecting refined ingredients and hydrogenated fats, while getting a lot more exercise. But according to a study in the *Archives of Internal Medicine*—a rigorous and respected journal—the great majority of us aren't taking that kind of care. Only 3 percent "consciously lead a healthy lifestyle that includes not smoking, exercising regularly, eating at least five daily servings of fruits and vegetables, and maintaining a healthy weight."[226] (See "Food as Medicine" on page 225) And while working out is routinely touted as the fountain of youth and longevity, according to the Harvard School of Public Health, less than 22 percent of us exercise regularly.[227]

To rekindle our interest, new findings suggest that regular exercise may do as much for our mood as a popular antidepressant. Breaking new ground, an investigation by Duke University psychologists found that over a four-month period of time, exercise and Zoloft (an antidepressant) worked equally well on mild, moderate, and severe depression.[228] I'd like to add that if exercise makes you feel worse it could be a symptom of adrenal fatigue, something we look for at the primary care practice where I work. If this is describing you, then take the saliva cortisol test found in the Resource Guide for this chapter and see your doctor for healthy solutions.

Given the statistics above, it's time to reconsider our approach. Clearly, knowledge alone isn't enough to reprogram our behavior. But pausing for a healing interlude can interrupt an automatic response—like reaching for that glazed donut or the remote—and reconnect us with the wise and knowing part of ourselves that recognizes that we matter enough to make sound choices. Responding positively to the needs of our body doesn't always involve activity, though. As you've seen before in the pages of this book, sometimes less is more. A study in *The Archives of Internal Medicine* recently made headlines when researchers discovered that people who take a nap at least three times a week for thirty minutes or more had a 37 percent lower risk of dying from a heart attack.[229] The drop in stress hormones may account for the results, but since we are not a nation of nap-takers (the study took place in Greece), we may want to reconsider the advantages of siestas.

Just Say No

Learning to care deeply for ourselves means moving beyond the "task" mentality popularized in our culture, where listing our accomplishments determines the quality of our day. We prove to ourselves that we really matter when we're willing to "just say no." Research reveals that survivors become very selective in their use of energy, know their limits, and respect them. Reflect on how would you respond to this statement—would you rate it true or false? "If someone I care about asks me to do a favor I'd rather not do, I'll do it anyway."[230] That statement is part of a questionnaire used by Lydia Temoshok, Ph.D., head of the U.S. Military's Behavioral Medicine Research Program on HIV/AIDS. A "true" response is associated with potentially negative immune effects. But don't worry—you may feel uneasy at first, but with practice and acting as if you have the right to say no, it gets easier with time. (One survivor, Susan Levitt joked, "I used to be a nice person!")

Now that you're convinced of the healing potential of saying "no," it's a great time to insert a paradox, something that seems to happen all the time in medicine. In what may seem like a perverse version of Simon Says, research also shows that contributing to others and being dedicated to a cause greater than yourself are hallmarks of survivors. The key difference seems to lie in the lack of familiarity with whom we're helping. This may not be so surprising when we think about it. Working in a soup kitchen can boost immunity; babysitting your six grandchildren when you don't feel like it can hurt you.

You might receive immune boosts like this through your work or gain a sense of mission in a hobby or volunteering for a cause you believe in. Psychologist and Professor of Bioethics Stephen G. Post, Ph.D., of Case Western Reserve University's School of Medicine has built his career on the scientific study of altruism, compassion, and service. His recent book, *Why Good Things Happen to Good People*, documents lower rates of illness and mortality among those who practice charitable works.[231] Along with Dr. Post, Allen Luks, a researcher who chronicles his findings in *The Healing Power of Doing Good*, has found that it's the process of helping, not the outcome, that's the healing factor.[232]

In tandem with altruism, studies in general link longevity to spirituality and a belief in something greater than yourself. Under the bleakest of conditions, individuals have found ways and means of doing good things for others. In concentration camps, meager rations were shared with the sick and the dying. And in nearly impossible situations, sharing the underlying meaning magnifies it. One woman who lived half her life in an iron lung never missed an opportunity to share the purpose and meaning she had found in life.

Information like this, though, can be frustrating under certain circumstances. Some have confided that the illness has robbed them of the energy to do what they enjoy, compromising their commitment to themselves and the opportunity to lend a helping hand to others. It can be comforting to keep in mind that when we are ill the cells of the immune system send out messenger molecules that travel back to the brain, producing chemical reactions that motivate us to rest. Very different from laziness, it is actually a heightened state of activity that harnesses resources for the healing process.

Metta

In this setting, commitment to yourself most resembles *metta*, a Pali word translated best as loving-kindness. In her book, *Lovingkindness: The Revolutionary Art of Happiness*, Sharon Salzburg defines loving-kindness as compassion, forgiveness, and love without judgment, along with our willingness to accept even unpleasant things as they are.[233] Metta is often challenged when we are faced with serious illness, where the body becomes the battlefield. At times we may feel alienated from our bodies—resentful of the pain and suffering—and so deny ourselves the understanding and compassion we might easily offer another. But we can only truly offer someone else what we have first given to ourselves. Sending metta to the aspects of ourselves that we have been struggling with is a wonderful way of learning to see through the eyes of compassion.

One of the most profound examples of metta is the story of Evy McDonald after she was diagnosed with amyotrophic lateral sclerosis (ALS), or Lou Gehrig's disease. Dr. Siegel tells the story in this excerpt from his book:

> She was told by her neurologist, "Evy, you have six to twelve months to live. If you want to do something nice, leave your body to science." That afternoon she was fired from her job as a nurse, because she had been out sick so much, and that evening she discovered that her apartment had been broken into and all her valuables stolen. At that point, she decided that her doctor's advice sounded pretty good.
>
> Evy knew that her journey would have to begin with an acceptance of her own body, which she had always hated, and in an article she wrote she describes how she accomplished that first step toward self-love:
>
> "There I sat in front of a mirror in my wheelchair. In the six months since I'd been diagnosed as having ALS, my once firm, strong muscles had wasted away into flaccid, useless ones. I was dying from a particularly rapid form of this incurable disease and had, at best, six more months to live. I looked with disgust at my deteriorating body. I hated it...
>
> As the hours of my day were now relegated to sitting alone in my wheelchair, I began to observe rather than react to my thoughts....
>
> As I sat in my wheelchair, six months from death, a single, passionate desire pressed to the front of my mind. In my last months of life I wanted to experience unconditional love. I wanted to know that sweetness.

But how could I even hope to realize that goal if I couldn't accept my own body?...

The first step was to notice and write down how many negative thoughts I had about my body in the course of each day, and how many positive ones. When I saw the huge preponderance of negative thoughts on the paper, I was forced to confront the degree of hatred I had for my body.

To counter this habitual and ingrained negativity, every day I singled out one aspect of my physical body that was acceptable to me, no matter how small. Next, I'd use that item to begin the rewriting. Every negative thought would be followed by a positive statement like "and my hair is truly pretty," or "I have lovely hands," or "my bright eyes and warm smile light up my face." Each day a different positive item would be added as each day, the rewriting continued.

I felt like a jigsaw puzzle being put back together; and when the last bit was in place, my mind shifted and saw the whole perfect picture. I couldn't pinpoint just when the shift occurred, but one day I noticed that I had no negative thoughts about my body. I could look in the mirror at my naked reflection and be honestly awed by its beauty. I was totally at peace, with a complete, unalterable acceptance of the way my body was—a bowl of jello in a wheelchair." [234]

Nearly a decade later I watched awestruck as Evy joined Bernie Siegel on stage in an inspirational address. Healing often begins with the compassionate acknowledgment of what we would like to be different. In a children's story by Shel Siverstein, a circle from which a large triangular wedge has been cut goes traveling around, rolling slowly because its "missing piece" prevents it from moving very fast. So along the way it's able to chat with butterflies and flowers, and to enjoy the sunshine. But being consumed with correcting its defect and becoming a perfect circle, it keeps looking for its missing piece. Finally, one day it finds a piece that fits exactly; it could finally be whole, with nothing missing! But now, as a perfect circle, it rolls along too fast to chat with butterflies or to notice the flowers. When it realizes how much has been lost, it stops, and leaves its missing piece by the side of the road and rolls on, slowly this time, once again savoring life, appreciating the "wholeness" offered by its missing piece.[235] Our missing piece becomes evident when we confront our limitations, and during times of illness, suffering, and loss. Yet it is the quality of our experiences, our limitations, and our wounds that enables us to connect profoundly and deeply with others.

At the cancer center we enjoyed a taste of this connectedness upon my return from Cape Cod, where I was one of four facilitators at ECaP leading a mind-body educational program for people with chronic illness. A participant from British Columbia picked up smooth, round pebbles on the shore and brought one back to each facilitator. We then respectively carried our stone back to our particular group at home. Members of our group in Atlanta experienced a unique sensation of connectedness as they held the stone, knowing that other people they would probably never meet had been thinking of them. They are linked by a powerful bond, a common thread of human experience.

But what if feelings of anger (at ourselves or others) get in the way of connecting deeply with those we care about? Often anger is a sign of engagement with life and can be a signal that something needs to change. Certainly the cancer studies by Levy, Temoshak, and Greer indicate that many people who recover become angry first. Anger can pave the path to establishing healthy boundaries and help us maintain our dignity and integrity in the face of life-altering disease. It's not the message of anger that poses the problem—it's what we do with it. It becomes an issue if we are overwhelmed by it, lashing out and alienating those we care about. Fortunately, there's help if anger is tripping us up. *The Dance of Anger* by Harriett Lerner, Ph.D., gives a fresh perspective if anger or resentment threatens our dealings with others. It's especially important because strong, positive relationships with others are essential to our well-being.

The feelings we hold about our bodies influence how we treat ourselves and sometimes how we conduct ourselves in intimate relationships. One woman, whose surgeon commented on the excellent results of her breast reconstruction, confided that she had not yet looked at her breast. It had been three years since reconstruction, but she could not bring herself to look at her body in a mirror. Ubiquitous but narrow images of beauty distort how we see ourselves. When I worked at Getting Well there was a poster on the wall of a woman in her sixties at the shore—waves in the background, sunlight behind her—with her arms stretched wide as if she were embracing the sky. She was beautiful and powerful, but she was also topless and clearly missing a breast. When walking into the room, men asked, "Why is that poster there?" As soon as someone pointed out the missing breast, the blushing man would grin and say, "Oh, of course, I get it." They just didn't see what was missing. But every woman who walked into that room noticed immediately. It never had to be pointed out.

The body dialogue in "Get Started Now" will help you tap into your own body's wisdom. You can use it any time you want more information about what you can do to heal.

Get Started Now: Body Dialogue

This exercise contains multiple areas of exploration: feelings of gratitude and appreciation for what is right, tuning into symptoms, identifying which behaviors get in your way, and locating an emotional state or way of being that may benefit you. Depending on your particular concern, you may choose to focus on one area and later revisit the other aspects of the exercise.

Revisit your healing corner of the world. Breathe in deeply and engage all your senses. When you are ready, focus on the sensation of breathing. You don't have to make anything happen, just feel the air moving in and out. Notice the rhythm of your breath. You may become aware of the way your clothing feels against your skin or the pressure on your body from the chair you might be sitting in. Perhaps there is tension or tightness; you might feel itchy or restless. Whatever you find, just let the sensations of your body come into your mind, whatever they may be. Acknowledge each feeling, while breathing in and out with conscious awareness.

Your lungs, vital to energy production, obtain oxygen from the atmosphere and bring it to millions of specialized cells. All without your conscious awareness, your breathing removes toxins and waste from your body and brings healing oxygen in. The beautiful filtering process even protects your heart. That great organ, pumping rhythmically, picks up the oxygen and delivers it to all the vessels of your body, contracting more than two billion times during a normal lifespan. With deep appreciation for this magnificent pump, move your attention down into your abdomen. On the right side is the largest organ in your body, your liver. This amazing organ filters toxins and chemicals, and aids in digestion. A powerhouse of function, your liver can even regenerate itself after losing as much as three quarters of its tissue. With a sense of admiration, imagine all that these great and vital organs accomplish. With gratitude, slowly move on to your spleen, your pancreas, and all the other organs and systems of your body, taking your time to appreciate and acknowledge all that they do for you.

Consider your joints, tendons, ligaments, muscles, and bones. And then your senses: the gifts of sight, smell, and hearing. Think deeply of all that they allow you to do and experience. All of these complex functions take place without effort or even awareness on your part—they just happen. Reflect on all that takes place—every minute of every day—and thank your body for all that is right with you. Notice how it feels to tune into your body on a deeper level. Consider now any symptoms you may have. Gently notice if there are any thoughts or behaviors that make some symptoms worse or better. Listen closely to your own intuitive awareness. Is there something you can do for your body to help it heal more completely? What can you do to make your body's job easier or reduce a burden of some kind?

Rather than reaching for a cup of coffee when you feel tired or popping an aspirin when you have a headache, ask yourself how you would feel if you could take a brisk walk in fresh air, or relax with some refreshing music, or even take a short nap. If it's not possible to do one of those things at that very moment, look for a way to bring it into play in another part of your day. Congratulate yourself for listening to your body.

Feel what it would be like to operate in your own best interest. What might that include? Are there positive feelings you would like to experience more often? If you had to choose just one, what would it be? In what way could you bring more of that quality into your life? In your mind's eye, see that happening now. Feel the peace, or the joy, or whatever it is you have chosen radiate throughout your being. And if it seems good to you, carry it with you, back to your healing place, and spend a moment in this serene setting enjoying the fullness of that sensation. When it seems right to you, again focus gently on your body, bringing your attention back to the chair or the place you happen to be. And filled with gratitude, stretch your arms wide with appreciation for all that is right with you.

Healing Connections

A great deal of evidence points to friendship as being a key player in longevity. A study reported in the *Journal of Epidemiology and Community Health* found that active friendships have a positive effect when it comes to "depression, self-efficacy, self-esteem, coping and morale, or a sense of personal control." (We know now how important control can be!) But more than a sense of well-being is at stake.

A ten-year study including more than one thousand people age seventy and up found that those who had a strong network of friends had a 22 percent lower mortality rate than those with few friends.[236] This may be cause for concern as recent headlines from a study conducted at Duke University reported that Americans have an average

> *There is no disease that kills people at the rate loneliness does... When disconnected people band together and develop ties, their health improves...Raising hope increases health; the attention of friends is an essential part of the brain's nutrition.*
>
> —ROBERT ORNSTEIN

of only two close friends—down from three in years past—with whom they can confide.[237] The high cost of loneliness is echoed in a small study of eighty-three healthy college students receiving flu shots at Carnegie Mellon University. Over a period of just four months, it was found that lonely students had lower concentrations of antibody production (indicative of a poorer immune response) along with poor sleep quality and quantity.[238]

Yet it may not be the number of close friends, per se, that proves to be so vital, but the quality and dimension of the support itself, as further evidence shows that having just one or two close friends greatly reduces the risk of dying from a stroke or heart attack. But here's the more telling discovery: in a Harvard study of more than fifty-six thousand women, the absence of a confidant was equal, as measured in physical decline, to being a heavy smoker and having the highest level of obesity! In this landmark investigation the death-dealing effects were avoided by having just one good friend.[239] If our intimate contacts are limited due to old conflicts or injuries, it may be time to start mending fences and stop holding grudges. A University of Miami study found that people who forgave a "close friend or family member who had treated them badly reported fewer aches and pains compared with those who kept sulking."[240] In *Living a Connected Life*,[241] clinical psychologist Kathleen Brehony takes a close look at the robust effect meaningful interactions—both giving and receiving—have on our health, and how we can maintain and strengthen the relationships we have.

In our transient and mobile society, though, the lack of close personal ties can leave us adrift. Widening our interpretation of how we see "family" is one way to meet that challenge. (This may be a good idea regardless, as the ten-year study mentioned above revealed that the health-protective effects of friendship didn't apply to relatives![242] Hmm…it reminds me of the British biographer and poet Hugh Kingsmill, who wrote, "Friends are God's apology for relatives.")

Redefining Family

Going outside the box in meeting your need for community, support, and understanding may mean becoming part of a group where you give and receive support, or seeing a professional therapist or counselor. There is no single right way to do this—or anything else. Trust and believe in yourself; act as if you're worth it, and ask for what you need. With help from your friends, community, group, or counselor, you too can receive the support and comfort you shouldn't be without.

A single parent with no family, Tom had three close friends who had never met each other. After his heart attack, he realized he would need help with housework, meals, and caring for his son. After discussing options, Tom's therapist arranged for a private meeting with the three friends and asked if they were willing to become his family during this difficult period. They each agreed and designed a schedule for meeting Tom's needs. In helping him through such a critical time, they were able to conquer some of their own fears and face their mortality in a meaningful way.

To benefit fully from the connections we have, we need to be specific. Expecting others to read our minds and divine our wishes perpetuates cycles of loneliness and resentment. One woman, a physical therapist, was recovering from surgery and needed help with her toddler and older child who had multiple handicaps. She emailed her community of friends and support people a list of all the things she needed help with for the next few months. For the most part people responded generously and lovingly. She said she knew she had to be explicit with her needs and not leave anything to chance and when people said "no," she had to come to grips with that, too. And she did.

Research indicates that we may gain a needed edge by joining a group. The feeling of belonging, in and of itself, may provide crucial protection. As you've read, evidence links higher than normal levels of cortisol (a stress hormone) to an increased risk of breast cancer, but for more than

one hundred participants with metastatic breast cancer a sense of belonging and feeling supported in a group setting were directly linked to
lower cortisol levels.[243] The researchers at Stanford University School
of Medicine concluded that a high quality of social support is associated
with lower cortisol levels, which indicate a healthier immune system.

Support groups like these help reduce the damaging effects of stress on
the individual as well as improve coping strategies. When Laura Leather-
wood, a group member at our cancer center, lost her daughter unexpectedly, Laura took in her daughter's child to raise, a seven-year-old boy.
Then one of Laura's sisters was brutally murdered by an ex-husband.
Soon after, Laura discovered that she had cirrhosis of the liver caused
by hepatitis C, which was then followed by a diagnosis of colon cancer. As she worked toward recovery, Laura continued to take care of the
household, raise her grandson, and support and care for another sister, a
woman with many physical and psychiatric problems. She set for herself
the goal of seeing her grandson enter college. Over time Laura completely recovered and even received the good news that the cirrhosis had
reversed itself. Laura was celebrating life, appreciating the extra time she
could share with her grandson. When he was close to graduating from
high school, Laura developed some mild digestive upsets and abdominal
swelling, but these symptoms were easily explained away. Soon, though,
exploratory surgery became necessary. This time, a rare, metastatic uterine sarcoma was found, and extensive surgery was performed.

Again on chemotherapy, Laura needed the safe harbor of the group
as she struggled with feelings that few in her community could understand. It is one of several reasons we offer an ongoing group format,
meeting once a month, for graduates of the six-week class. Although
Laura never again became cancer free, her last year was characterized
by the gentle grace that guided her life. Before she died she witnessed
her grandson enter college, exactly as she had wished eleven years earlier. Laura's legacy remains strong among the group members who have

been meeting monthly for more than twelve years now! As in the books mentioned earlier, Henry Dreher presents compelling evidence in *The Immune Power Personality*[244] that people who love and connect with others are more likely to survive a disease or a concentration camp. Survivors learn to ask for favors from friends and family, neighbors, and community, as well as seek professional help. One woman who always focused on giving or doing things for others said she never knew how much people cared about her until she learned to receive. The group you choose should offer a haven for your unique emotional needs and even provide practical physical help when possible. Skills can be taught. Victimization can be transformed into empowerment. All of which can affect our longevity. In a matched case control study, participants who attended six two-hour health psychology classes lived significantly longer than did their counterparts who did not participate. (None of the patients in the intervention group died, compared to 12 percent of the control group.[245]) For housebound folks or those in periods of recovery, online groups such as PatientsLikeMe offer a forum for sharing information and support.[246]

In addition to reaching out, connecting with others, and making their needs known, another interesting quality of survivors is that they don't resist change. If you were to walk into the Helen and Harry Gray Cancer Center in Hartford, Connecticut, you might notice a mobile structure slowly turning above you. Commissioned by the chief oncologist, Andrew Salner, it was designed to imitate life: no two moments are the same—the wheel of change is inevitable. Combating change can be like defying gravity—it can't be done, and attempting it can hurt you. Living in the past, or grieving over what might have been, short circuits the energy required for healing in the present. Being open to change is a sign of health, the opposite of desperately trying to maintain the status quo. If you're a resister of change, take heart! There is a powerful technology that firmly grounds you peacefully and realistically in the present and helps you accept changes in the future. It can also work wonders for your mind and body.

The Technology of Mindfulness

Scores of findings over the past ten years attest to the mental, emotional, and physical value of mindfulness[247]—another technology in your defense. Mindfulness has been shown to positively influence many conditions from irritable bowel syndrome to heart disease. This deceptively simple practice is one of the techniques, along with imagery, that researchers found to have a striking effect in preventing all manner of illness. The evidence is so strong that some insurance companies offer discounts to members who practice approved techniques.[248] Jon Kabat Zinn, creator of the mindfulness based stress reduction (MBSR) program at the University of Massachusetts Medical Center, has found that focusing on the present not only releases tension, but can reset the body's thermostat, assisting in regulating the autonomic nervous system.[249]

You have already seen how something as insubstantial as a thought or an image can alter the very structure of the brain. Before-and-after brain scans in experiments with patients suffering from obsessive compulsive disorder (OCD) reveal that just ten weeks of mindfulness training is as effective as standard drug therapy. The pivotal role of healing technologies such as mindfulness is reinforced by psychobiologist Ernest Rossi, linking it with "compassion, beneficence, serenity, forgiveness and gratitude."[250] In an experiment by Richard J. Davidson of the University of Wisconsin, twenty-five participants took a weekly class in mindfulness meditation for a total of eight weeks. In addition, participants were instructed to practice the technique on their own for one hour a day, six days a week. At the conclusion of the eight weeks, the meditation group and nineteen control subjects received a flu vaccine. The meditators not only had higher levels of protective antibodies, but also had increased activity in parts of the brain associated with positive emotion. The effects were still present when participants were tested again, four months later.[251]

You naturally experience mindfulness when you are deeply in tune with nature, meditating on the sound of waves on the water or watching the clouds go by. But it's the efficiency of mindfulness that captures my interest. In chapter 6 I alluded to a technique that could help transform the tedious and unavoidable to-do items on your list. Through the effects of mindfulness almost any activity can be turned into a meditative one. Without changing your activities or the rhythm of your day, by gently returning your attention mindfully to whatever you're doing, you reap the rewards. By way of illustration, let's say that after work I'm fighting rush hour traffic and realize that I'm going to be behind for the rest of my evening commitments. Arriving home, there's barely enough time to throw dinner together and greet my husband before I jump back in the car and whoosh off to a night class. In this scenario, no matter what I'm doing, I'm racing through one activity and scrambling through another. With mindfulness on my side, the very same activities—driving, making dinner, seeing my husband, leaving the house—take on a restorative, meditative quality. In traffic, I might find myself grateful that I'm in an air-conditioned automobile, listening to music in stereo. At home chopping celery, I might meditate on what an unusual vegetable celery really is—it's crisp but stringy. Rather than mindlessly unloading the dishwasher and setting the table, I might choose to focus on how cool it is that I can take out smooth, clean plates and feel grateful that I have someone to share the meal with.

By focusing solely on one thing at a time in a nonjudgmental, meditative way, by the time I leave for my evening class, I'm feeling peaceful, present, and refreshed. The advantages even spill over into the creative problem-solving arena. In a presentation I attended, Harvard professor and author of *Mindfulness* Ellen Langer recommended that we not learn anything so well that we can do it absent mindedly—whether we are gardening, cooking, painting, or drawing—because we can lose the fresh perspective that invites us to incorporate what we've learned into unrelated situations and activities.

Experiment with mindfulness as you move through your day. While the nature of mind is to wander, gently bringing your attention back to the present fights forward thinking—a major cause of hurry and worry, not to mention stress hormones and unhappiness—and grounds you in gratitude for the prosaic details of everyday life. When we find ourselves concerned about the future or fretting about the past, mindfulness anchors us firmly in the present. With this mindset it's easier to cultivate an appreciative spirit, which in turn counteracts any lingering sense of vigilance and turmoil.

In a workshop I attended, writer and researcher Janet Quinn, Ph.D., told the story of a young man dying of HIV/AIDS back in the day before protease inhibitors. When I asked if the account was written anywhere she answered "just in my heart," and gave me permission to share it with you. One day in particular stands out in Janet's mind. When they met together, the young man rocked silently in his chair for a moment and then mindfully related the events of his morning—the glint of the sun shining on the dew when he went out to get the paper and the sweet taste of the orange juice. As he sat on the porch to read he marveled at the songs of the birds. He wasn't in denial about dying nor was he focused on it; rather, he was searching out the beauty in each and every moment. Absorbing the details. Savoring the experience. What eloquent appreciation of the sensory world that we often take for granted! All of our busy-ness can consume us with a false sense of importance. The young man's story gives us cause to pause and reflect—in all our hurry and worry—whether we are missing out on living. It breaks our perception of what winning, acquiring, and achieving really mean, and shows us how exquisite our moment-to-moment existence can be when we're mindfully living in the present.

In confiding a past suicide attempt, a client said that before taking enough pills to render her unconscious for five days, she drove to McDonald's and slowly savored a Big Mac, some fries, and a milkshake. She said it was so delicious, made so by knowing she'd never have it again. (Who knows—maybe that "last supper" saved her life by preventing the complete absorption of the toxic overload!) The bigger lesson is, how much of our depression or suffering could be alleviated by the exquisite focus and appreciation of the moment?

Scores of findings say it can do that and more (see endnotes on mindfulness in this chapter). According to the evidence, mindfulness also helps with emotional control and equilibrium, something that can be compromised if you have a high ACE score (Adverse Childhood Experience Study discussed in chapter 7). Observing, rather than reacting to, our thoughts can keep us from becoming overwhelmed by our feelings. Being present enriches our experience of the moment but also opens the door to alternative possibilities that we might have overlooked.

> *Expecting fairness in life is a gigantic energy waster. The fact is, once you're done with the fairness hang-up, you can really make serious progress.*
>
> —ROLAND NOLEN

The Reluctant Hero

When I think about putting the six-week program into long-term practice I am reminded of Chad. Covert operations as a Navy Seal led him to dangerous locales and threatening conditions. But he faced none so menacing as what was uncovered in a routine blood test. By cold rote, the physician spared no detail about what he could expect with incurable chronic myelogenous leukemia (CML). Even with a bone marrow transplant—the gold standard of treatment for CML—he had a fifty-fifty chance of survival. Without a transplant, under the best of conditions, he could hope to see his daughter, now in kindergarten, enter third grade.

Reeling from the fierce and unyielding prognosis, Chad's first order of business was a second opinion. Then a third. After that a fourth and a fifth. He explained, "I was in a bit of denial—like checking a lottery ticket a couple of times to make sure you don't have any of the winning numbers." Facing his new reality, he launched a different kind of search—not for a clean bill of health, but for the kind of doctor he could trust to partner him in the biggest challenge of his life. He chose two: a CML specialist at MD Anderson Cancer Center in Houston, Texas, and an Atlanta oncologist, Gerry Goldklang, who would provide local support. Together they chose to view his prognosis as unpredictable rather than absolute, and the bone marrow drives began.

In the meantime, Chad began to search for those things he could control, such as diet and exercise. He participated in my six-week class and scrutinized his beliefs, practiced imagery and expressive writing, and drew a series of pictures of himself and his treatment that I still have today. Chad eagerly gathered new skills and a different kind of confidence. When one treatment became ineffective, he tried another. The bone marrow drives continued, but still without a match. Staying alive until there was a cure became his mantra. Participating in various clinical trials at MD Anderson demanded four to six trips a year, sometimes requiring stays as long as a month at a time. While Interferon was the standard drug therapy for CML, MD Anderson was more aggressive with the dose. Despite side effects, Chad stayed fit and volunteered with the Leukemia Society of America, raising money for research by running in long-distant marathons in Alaska and biking over a hundred miles in Tucson, Arizona.

After a three-year national search of thousands and thousands of potential bone marrow donors the search was concluded without a match being found. Practicing mindfulness, Chad focused on the life he had now with his wife and daughter. Taking nothing for granted, he anchored himself firmly in the present—while planning for the future—and filled his life with meaning and purpose. Each year he reviewed his short and long-term wish list and made plans to see, do, learn, and experience whatever was on his list. When Chad passed the outermost limit of his prognosis, he saw his daughter finish third grade. And then fourth grade. Then fifth. Without a bone marrow transplant, without a recognized viable therapy, Chad was beating the odds. Trial after clinical trial with experimental treatments, Chad would not relinquish hope.

Unbeknownst to Chad though, on one of those trips to Texas (flying compliments of Corporate Angels), he became the second person to receive Gleevec, the drug that would become, years later, the cure for chronic myelogenous leukemia. The trial included a nine-week stay for twenty people at three locations: California, Oregon, and Texas. Because of extraordinary results, in April of 2001 Gleevec received early FDA approval and was opened to the public. As I write these words, it has been thirteen years since Chad was told that without a bone marrow transplant he would die. Last year Chad and his wife drove their daughter to Yale University for her freshman year. He is now the longest living person on Gleevec.

While Chad didn't deny the reality of his diagnosis, he defied the prognosis. Viewing it as a turning point, rather than an end point, he took control and changed physicians. He employed belief in treatments and in his doctors. Still, despite their healing partnership, he didn't give his power away to either his doctor or the clinical trial, but took responsibility for what he could change or control. Chad remained absolutely committed to himself and while actively cultivating ethical hope, he never denied his own mortality, but all the while kept the number nine bus etched firmly in his consciousness.

May you, too, mindfully breathe and seek wonder, fascination, and purpose as you live connected to and aware of all that you hold dear. The next chapter reveals three essential questions that will help keep you on track.

❧

FOOD AS MEDICINE

With all the diet and nutrition information available it's no wonder the question of supplements comes up frequently in the six-week class. Certain herbs and nutrients, while perhaps beneficial on their own, can interfere with or result in serious side effects when taken with certain medications, chemotherapies, and radiation therapy. Nutritious, whole foods, however, don't carry this risk. For effective repair whole vitamin complexes—as they exist in nature—are ideal as they are readily absorbed and utilized by the body.

A leader in this area is oncologist James Gordon, founder of the Center for Mind-Body Medicine in Washington, D.C., who offers a special educational program for physicians and clinicians entitled Food as Medicine. That is one reason why the only supplement routinely recommended by Dr. Gerry Goldklang at Georgia Cancer Treatment Center is Juice Plus. It doesn't interfere with medical treatment because it's just food—something your body recognizes and knows what to do with!

Bioavailability is key:

Several university studies have concluded that Juice Plus effectively increases plasma levels of antioxidants and other phytonutrients.

Clinical research has shown lipid peroxides (an indicator of oxidative stress), homocysteine levels, and even DNA damage were reduced by taking Juice Plus.

A study published in the *Journal of the American College of Cardiology* demonstrated that its phytonutrients negated the arterial constriction that typically occurs after eating a high fat meal.

The Journal of Integrative Medicine published a study showing this simple supplement increased T-cell and NK cell activity—critical to healthy immune function. See the research tab of their website for more.

Probiotics are another restorative aid that can help your immune system return to a healthy state. The vital and beneficial bacteria that reside in your gut perform too many priceless services to name here. But antibiotics and other treatments can drastically reduce their number, leaving you vulnerable to diarrhea and all sorts of unpleasant side effects. The good news is that a variety of these healthy bacteria can protect and even repair the lining of your intestines, which in turn lightens the load on your liver. (And don't forget how important the gut is to your immune system!) Probiotics naturally occur in buttermilk and yogurt (as long as it contains viable cultures), but you can also find a ready-made supply at your local health food store.

Lastly, the American Heart Association recommends an essential fatty acid found in cold-water fish like salmon, mackerel, and sardines as well as in nuts and flax seed. Omega-3, famous for its anti-inflammatory effects, is also good for your brain and is reported to be an effective adjunct in the treatment of some types of depression. If your diet isn't rich in cold-water fish or you are concerned about its mercury content then a mercury-free fish oil supplement may be in order.

Other specific recommendations by your doctor or a knowledgeable nutritionist can help speed your recovery and bring your body back into balance. To meet this need at the Cancer Center, we host occasional seminars conducted by a clinical nutritionist or a physician schooled in integrative or functional medicine. You may benefit from an individual consultation yourself. See the Resource Guide for more.

Week Six

⊰ 9 ⊱

The Biology of Belief: Remapping Your Brain with Cognitive Insight

We are disturbed not by events, but by the views that we take of them.
—EPICTETUS, FIRST CENTURY GREEK PHILOSOPHER

My husband was driving around the airport while I dashed inside to pick up our airline tickets. Leaving the terminal, I quickly spotted the car. Opening the door, I stared at the cassette tapes and CDs scattered on the front seat. They didn't look familiar. Confused but pushing a few aside anyway, I began to sit down and close the door. Then I looked up at the startled stranger in the driver's seat. We both jumped. I was so certain that this was my car that I almost asked him what he had done with my husband. Of course, my mindlessness hit me and—between giggles—I apologized profusely, explaining that my husband had a car exactly like his. After the man had picked up his family they drove by, all waving with big grins. If only all our blind assumptions were so quickly corrected!

Through the Looking Glass

Like when we look into a fun house mirror at a carnival, we can easily lose our balance if our perception is distorted. Because our biology readily responds to our beliefs, our healing potential can be stymied not only by stress hormones, but by self-limiting thinking and irrational thoughts. When beating the odds, our lens of perception needs to be crystal clear. Polishing that lens means taking a closer look at how we learn to see.

By a miracle of technology, babies born blind today from congenital cataracts can have their vision restored through a surgical procedure. But the same operation is no magic bullet when performed on adults who are blind since birth. If an infant is unable to see, the visual cortex begins recruiting other systems to compensate, such as hearing (called cross-modal plasticity). As a result, those adults who suddenly have their sight restored are pitched into an agonizing orbit of spinning lights and colors. Unable to recognize objects without touching them, it is years before they truly learn how to see. In an iconic and horrible experiment, kittens were blindfolded at birth and when their blindfolds were removed they were unable to see even though there were no physical abnormalities. The brains of the blind infants and kittens were untrained in the rules of seeing—rules we didn't even know existed, but learned nonetheless in childhood. Although we may have our sight intact, some of these rules still act as a filter and distort our perception of reality.

Our individual perspective is shaped, not only by our family of origin, but by the prevailing views of our particular society as a whole. As outrageous as it seems today, it was once considered heretical to conceive that the earth was not the center of the universe. Equally outrageous, physicians went from the morgue to the maternity ward without washing their hands because the idea that germs carried disease seemed a great flight of fancy. In fact, in the 1840s when Dr. Ignaz Semmelweis began promoting the idea that physicians were killing mothers by delivering babies after handling cadavers without washing their hands, he was dismissed from the hospital where he was employed, shunned, and eventually committed to a psychiatric asylum.[252] But where would we be today if no one took the risk of challenging the prevailing dogma or paused to ask, "Is it really so?"

The trap of traditional thinking may be safe—but it's also self-limiting. There may be no better example of how belief affects the body than the well-researched yet still mysterious placebo effect that you read about in chapter 2. Operative in almost every condition known to man, it's the measurable, medicinal result of belief in action, which is so reliable and predictable that most every drug in your medicine cabinet has been tested in trials against it by use of the humble sugar pill. A classic example of the placebo effect comes from a study conducted in 1950 using syrup of ipecac.[253] If you're a parent—or a bulimic—you probably know that it is a powerful emetic (something that makes you throw up). But in this rather bold study, Dr. Stewart Wolf gave it to women who were already nauseous from extreme morning sickness, telling them it would settle their stomachs. And it did.

How We Know: Hard Evidence for Positive Thinking

Just as what we believe about a pill or a potion can affect complicated body processes, the way we think and explain things to ourselves can be used to predict our longevity. While positive thinking is somewhat of a cliché in mind-body work, credible and increasing evidence points to positive affect (or emotion) as a major player in chronic illness. Considering all the factors beyond our control—where and how we grew up for example—it can come as a relief to discover that attitude can be a stronger influence on mortality than smoking history and sociodemographic variables. (For a refresher on the true definition of a positive attitude see "The Myth of the Positive Attitude" under Popular Pitfalls in chapter 2.)

A case in point is a 2008 study of diabetics that found qualities such as hope, happiness, and life enjoyment to be "significantly associated" with a lower risk of dying from all causes.[254] (Since diabetes is the sixth leading cause of death in the United States, studies like this make an impression.) Similar findings are reported for folks suffering from rheumatoid arthritis, hypertension, and fibromyalgia.[255] The benefits hold true even for those without a chronic illness. The same researchers, from the University of California at San Francisco, also examined more than two thousand healthy people. For those aged sixty-five and older, the very same qualities—hope, happiness, and life enjoyment—were associated with a significantly reduced risk of mortality from all causes.[256] Curiously, this did not apply to those younger than sixty- five. Although attitude didn't predict the health status of younger people in the above case, another study shows it *can* predict how well you age. In this project, despite the fact that most of the five hundred participants had some sort of illness or disability, Dr. Dilip Jeste of the University of California at San Diego determined it was "optimism and effective coping styles" that were "more important to aging successfully than traditional measures of health and wellness." He concludes, "These findings suggest that physical health is not the best indicator of successful aging—attitude is."[257]

In the past, some studies have linked optimism to healthy behaviors, counting in part for at least some of the effects. But a recent Harvard study proved otherwise. Over a thousand healthy men with no known health conditions were carefully evaluated for qualities of optimism and pessimism. After a ten-year follow up researchers found that the optimists had half the risk of coronary artery disease than the pessimists, even after smoking history and other traditional risk factors were accounted for.[258]

Particularly persuasive are findings reported in "Does How You Do Depend on How You Think You'll Do?" from the *Canadian Medical Association Journal,* which examines the relationship between our expectations for recovery and outcome. In this careful analysis of the research, fifteen out of sixteen well-designed studies demonstrate a strong graded relationship between belief and recovery. Patients who had positive expectations had better health outcomes overall.[259]

Echoing these findings is Dr. Erik Giltay, lead investigator in a fifteen-year study of optimism and pessimism in the Netherlands. In this project, researchers followed more than five hundred men without existing heart problems, between the ages of sixty-four and eighty-four. Over a fifteen-year period, the men took quizzes on optimism while their health and other factors were evaluated. The result? Optimistic men were an amazing 55 percent less likely to die of all causes and 23 percent less likely to die from heart problems than the pessimists![260] Dr. Erik Giltay, M.D., Ph.D., has generously given permission for you to take the quiz (published in the Archives of Internal Medicine) used in the study and quickly gauge your own optimism quotient.

Get Started Now: The Optimism Quiz

Rate each of the four statements: Fully Agree, Partially Agree, Don't Agree, Don't Know

1. I still expect much from life.
2. I do not look forward to what lies ahead for me in the years to come.
3. My days seem to be passing slowly.
4. I am still full of plans.

Scoring guidelines:

Statement number 1: Fully agree—2 points. Partially agree or Don't Know—1 point, Don't Agree—0 points

Statement number 2: Fully agree—0 points. Partially agree or Don't Know—1 point, Don't Agree—2 points.

Statement number 3: Fully agree—0 points. Partially agree or Don't know—1 point, Don't Agree—2 points.

Statement number 4: Fully agree—2 points. Partially agree or Don't know—1 point, Don't Agree—0 points.

The higher your score, the more optimistic you're feeling.

We can speculate on the findings, but at this point they are creating ripples in an intense debate that we'll get to in a moment. At the heart of the issue is a project that's been ongoing for over half a century. Returning from World War II, two hundred sixty-eight Harvard graduates were interviewed and followed with physical exams every five years. Decades later, the astonishing data revealed that the way the young men explained bad events at age twenty-five predicted their health and quality of life twenty to thirty-five years later! Driving the point home is an equally strong study conducted by the Mayo Clinic that tracked more than eight hundred patients over a thirty-year period, and established a solid link between higher levels of optimism and lower mortality rates.[261]

These investigations, though, are incredibly complex. Part of the difficulty in studying attitude and aging is the huge degree of external factors that can confound results—such as marital status, number of children, occupation, excessive alcohol intake, and socioeconomic factors. Complicating matters further, in an aging population essential information may not be recalled accurately, particularly in those with dementia or Alzheimer's. So Dr. David Snowdon, epidemiologist and professor of neurology, along with his colleagues at the University of Kentucky, decided that nuns who entered convent life over sixty years ago would make ideal subjects.[262] It was a brilliant move. In convent life most of those variables would disappear. What's more, when they entered the convent as young women they completed detailed autobiographical statements and had yearly checkups thereafter. Together these records could provide a rich tapestry of valuable clinical data. Sophisticated computer analysis, specially designed for the task, would scrutinize layers of thinking patterns and collate the information with decades of annual exams.

These autobiographical statements—and the brains of the nuns (most of which are being examined after their deaths)—hold so much potential for researchers that over five million tax dollars, not counting private donations, have been shuttled to the National Institute on Aging. Today, nearly seven hundred women over seventy-five years old are being studied. Like the Rosetta Stone, every detail of the nuns' statements has been coded, classified, and compared to their clinical data and health history. Looking for clues to explain significant differences in longevity and vitality, researchers found that the greater the number of positive emotions, the lower the risk of disability and mortality later in life. There is another crucial finding, but we'll get to that soon. In the meantime, let's take a closer look at optimism and its dark side, pessimism.

The Bless in the Mess

My father grew up poor in the South. Selling boiled peanuts on the street corner and recording tobacco sales in a warehouse, he slept on a cot in the hall while his three sisters shared the only available bedroom. As an adult, he became an expert at missile configuration (pioneering the science proving missiles didn't need wings) and in his early thirties worked with the Apollo program. With all the childhood lectures he gave my brother and me on the power of a positive attitude, I can only surmise that my dad felt there was an awful lot of complaining going on for two kids who had their own bedrooms.

He loved to make his point with the following joke: A man had twin sons. One son was a true optimist—nothing had influenced him to have a more balanced and realistic perspective of life. The other son was a serious pessimist and nothing seemed to help him to have a more positive outlook. Their extreme natures weighed heavily on their father, so one day he came up with a plan he felt certain would cure the two boys. For the pessimist, he filled an entire room with a dazzling array of toys, games, sweets, and every imaginable kind of treat. Then he locked the boy in the room for the day. "There!" thought the father, "Even he can find nothing negative about that room." The second room he filled with manure and locked the optimist in it for the day. "There!" he thought, "Even he can find nothing good about this room."

Pleased with his plan and imagining his two sons emerging from his experiment with a more balanced perspective, he went to the pessimist's room at the end of the day and opened the door. There he sat, crying in the middle of the room, toys untouched, sweets uneaten, games not played with. "What," the father cried, "could you possibly find wrong with any of these wonderful things?!" Sobbing heavily the boy replied, "The toys—they may break. And if I leave one in the rain it will rust. And the games—I may lose a piece if I play with them. And the sweets—if I eat too many I will get sick. It's just too sad, too sad." Distressed, the father left the room thinking: Surely I will be successful with my other son! Entering the second room he sees the optimist happily and excitedly shoveling manure. "What," the father cried, "could you possibly find good about a room full of manure?!" "Dad," the boy replied, "with all this manure, there's gotta be a pony in here somewhere!"

Some researchers may side with the frustrated father, as a few studies hint at a genetic set-point to happiness and optimism. Dr. Giltay shared with me that given the current research, he believes it's probably hard to improve an individual's level of optimism through psychotherapy. One of the reasons for this is that word choice (the words we use are identifiers or clues of how we think) is thought to be stable over a lifetime. But increasingly that view is being challenged. A revolutionary computer program designed to analyze word choice, tone, and pattern (including the connotations of the word) suggests otherwise. In a project spearheaded by Dr. Pennebaker, whom you met in chapter 7, this technology (called Linguistic Inquiry and Word Count, or LIWC) was used to determine which features of word choice might predict health and other factors. A combined analysis of forty-five different studies, with thousands of participants from three different countries, revealed that word choice was not stable over time. Running counter to popular belief, researchers found that people in general get more positive, even happier, as they age, not crankier, and that they use more positive words than when they were younger.[263] Further confounding conventional views, aging was associated with an *increase* in complex words and sentences. (You're not getting older, you're getting smarter!)

With conflicting studies, the debate is a hot one, with researchers as polarized as the concepts themselves. Extreme views of optimism and pessimism—as in the joke about the twins—add to some of the confusion. Making a departure from clichés and giving us a nuanced view of optimism is Dr. Martin Seligman, professor, author, and pioneer of the positive psychology movement. His solid research teases out various facets of optimism and helps us see the dimensions around positive thinking.[264]

For example, meeting me in person, you might label me optimistic, and you would be right—to a degree. As it happens, Atlanta, Georgia, lies on a fault line and unlike just about every single one of my friends, I happen to have earthquake insurance. Given that we've only had a few exceptionally mild tremors, this may be either paranoid or pessimistic, but no one has called me Henny Penny yet (at least not to my face). Either way, I've taken what I believe to be a proactive stance so I can forget about it and not worry about whether the sky is falling. Planning for a disaster may knock a few points off my total optimism scale, but it also lowers my anxiety. For me, that's a safe trade.

Other overtones of optimism are broken down further. As it turns out, we could be optimistic when our car washing business is booming and then pessimistically blame ourselves when business slacks off during monsoon season. There are ratios and perspectives involved. Coming up, you'll have a chance to participate in the debate and discover for yourself where you stand on the topic. Until then, you might like knowing that optimism, after all, does not mean that you need to convince yourself that you enjoy a job you hate! But it does mean evaluating what is and isn't working and deciding if it is in your best interest to make an adjustment. Moving beyond black and white, all or nothing thinking helps us look for realistic ways of upgrading our thinking style—and according to Dr. Seligman, our happiness as well. But while we're waiting for all the evidence to come in, one thing is clear: we have choices. Choices, as Dee Brigham, director of Getting Well, said, in how we see our world and in how we see our disease.

Get Started Now: Rate Your Attitude

Dr. Seligman has made a career of studying optimism and believes you can raise the level of your happiness with appropriate thought processes. To get started, take the free tests at www.authentichappiness.org to quickly determine your thinking and planning style and identify specific areas where you may benefit from a tune-up. Everything is automatically scored and your results are instantly available. After practicing with some of the tools to increase happiness, track your results by retaking the tests to see where you've upgraded your attitude. Your anonymity is protected, and your results will add to the research. Best of all, you can use the evidence you collect on yourself to take part in the debate.

Conflicting studies aside, tempers flare for yet another reason. Blasting the positive psychology movement, critics refer to it as the "tyranny" of positive thinking. If you've read the chapters that precede this one then you know I'm not prescribing Pollyanna platitudes, but rather seeking aspects of perception and thought that can serve us in our darkest hours. A shift in our thinking can help us overcome challenges we might not have thought possible.

In graduate school, one of my faculty advisors—Dr. Anne Webster, director of Harvard's mind-body medicine program for cancer and HIV—shared the story of a young man she worked with who was dying. He and his wife wanted to make a video of his playtime with their two-year-old son, something the boy could treasure when he was older. Weak and on pain medication, the young father would save every bit of energy he had in order to play with his son for a few minutes each day. But as soon as the camera would start to roll, he would sob. An already tragic and tender moment was made all the more gut wrenching by the inability to make the keepsake. After he shared his dilemma with Dr. Webster, she suggested that a subtle change in thinking would help him reach his goal. When the tears began, the man would ask himself, "Is this helping me now?" By asking that simple question he was able to put aside his grief for that moment in time, and over the course of his last few weeks of life, make the video he wished for his son.

Reframing a tragic situation or tuning up an unproductive worldview buffers some of the crushing effects of the calamities that can befall us. Questioning our automatic assumptions builds a repertoire of positive self-beliefs that support us during periods of crisis and change.

Change Your Mind, Change Your Brain

New technology shows we can remodel and reshape the brain itself. As discoveries mount, one of the biggest surprises for scientists—and stroke victims—is the degree of plasticity, or flexibility, the brain has. simply put, our brain is much more capable of recovering from dramatic and catastrophic injuries than ever imagined.

Your mind will be like its habitual thoughts: for the soul becomes dyed with the color of its thoughts.

—MARCUS AURELIUS

This is because the brain is constantly refining itself by promoting certain neurochemical pathways or circuits and trimming off old pathways that are either not being used or are no longer beneficial.

When you're inspired, the resulting new way of thinking virtually remaps your brain. Dr. Ernest Rossi explains that when a particular area of the brain is stimulated by novelty or enrichment, that region actually grows more neurons (called neurogenesis). "There are 2,100,000,000,000,000 connections among the nerve cells of the brain... This means that there are more possible mental states in each person's brain than there are atoms in the known universe."[265] Rossi has a personal side to the story when he talks about neurogenesis, the regeneration of neuronal tissue in the brain. When I attended his workshop on the subject, I discovered that he had suffered a stroke a few months prior. What he knew about regeneration kept him on task with the tedious aspects of his physical therapy, and there he was before us, speaking and moving well, his presence underscoring the wonders of brain plasticity even more than his beautiful slides, graphs, and other hard data.

The way we perceive or interpret our situation can degrade or restore, and the words we choose and the way we talk to ourselves can hurt or heal, affecting the very matter of the brain itself. Scans reveal that as we shift gears emotionally, a corresponding area of the brain lights up. Techniques that help us break out of a negative belief system rewire the brain's circuitry so that we can make necessary changes for a happier life and greater well-being. (By the way, the mindful awareness you read about in the previous chapter has also been shown to promote brain plasticity as well.)

The ultimate benefit for us in the here-and-now is that this powerful natural mechanism can be used in a more direct and intentional way in daily life to promote improvement in brain function. And immunity. Earlier, I promised to share another discovery from the nun study with you. What researchers noticed first was the healthiest nuns' autobiographical statements (written when they first entered the convent) were "idea dense," in contrast to the less grammatically complex ones, as seen in the nuns who developed Alzheimer's. Supporting this idea is a crucial finding from Dr. Pennebaker's LIWC program. In this computerized analysis of journal entries, those using the most cognitive words, such as *because* or *reason*, and insight words such as *realize* or *understand*, enjoyed better health overall. Specifically, folks using these word categories made fewer doctor visits for illness than the other group. While we'll have to wait for all aspects of the research to be analyzed, results so far reflect on the benefits of enriching our lives, which includes regularly learning new things.

The largest study of centenarians in the world bears this out. A 2006 study of thirty-two centenarians found almost all to be living independently or requiring minimal assistance.[266] Smashing stereotypes of aging, they were walking, biking, playing golf, and exercising their brains with stimulating mental activity such as reading, painting, or playing a musical instrument or a computer game. If your family tree isn't loaded with centenarians, there's hope. A report in the *Archives of General Psychiatry* indicates that simply having a predisposition toward optimism provided a survival benefit in elderly subjects otherwise predicted to have relatively short lives.[267]

Unplug from Negative Thinking

Our silent intentions carry weight and the ability to shape our future. Like a subliminal Hollywood script, we act out our belief system. If our belief is, "Bad things always happen to me," how many times will we unconsciously create the conditions that bring about misfortune? Of course, we all experience misfortune and life *is* unfair. The title of a well-known book isn't *If Bad Things Happen to Good People*, it's

> *Man is the only animal that laughs and weeps, for he is the only animal that is struck with the difference between what things are, and what they ought to be.*
>
> —WILLIAM HAZLITT

When.[268] But in between the unfair and the misfortune lies a large universe of opportunities—for hope, for mystery.

Unfortunately, our responses are often automatic. As we no longer notice ingrained patterns we can all too easily become lost in a frame of reference that is no longer beneficial. Like a well-traveled superhighway, the roads of familiar thinking are smooth and well lit. We're riding in comfort, the signs are easy to read; we even feel safe. Changing our thinking is like going off-roading: it's rough and rowdy work, plowing across unmarked territory, mowing down brush and brambles. The familiar route may feel much more comfortable, even if you're going in the wrong direction! But with a map (tools for positive thinking) and a great vehicle (your brain), your crooked thinking will soon be smoothed out, new neuronal connections will form, the very matter of your brain will accommodate this new line of thinking, and you'll be traveling safely and comfortably again. Since our beliefs can become a bit of a self-fulfilling prophecy, becoming crystal clear on exactly what they are puts us back in control.

Dr. Kathleen Brehony shared a secret of her golf game based on this idea. "I can hit 190 yard drives (sometimes) except when I am going over water. Then I splash in even though it was only 125 yards to clear it! Now I just say, 'What water?' And if I can make myself belief there is no water, I clear it easily." Capturing our fleeting thoughts, though, may not be as easy as it sounds. We can be well into a feeling before we realize it and may not be able to pinpoint the particular thought that produced the feeling. It's worth pursuing. Pennebaker writes, "there is reason to believe that when people transform their feelings and thoughts about personally upsetting experiences into language, their physical and mental health often improve."[269] With practice we can detect our style of thinking—and make adjustments accordingly—and feel happier overall as a result.

The easiest way to begin is by taking notes on the way you talk to yourself. Listen closely to the words you say to yourself as you move through your day—when you make a mistake, feel discouraged, or just happen to be running late for an appointment. Don't react; just observe the typical train of thoughts that travel through your mind during the day. Then gently respond to your thinking style with nonjudgmental self-awareness. If your silent self-talk is sabotaging your self-worth, start by noticing and then substituting supportive statements. For example, if you catch yourself making self-critical remarks, try a neutral phrase such as, "There it is again," or "How interesting." Then replace the contaminated thought with something heartening and reassuring.

At this point, people usually wonder what they're supposed to do with their list of resolutions or other things that they feel they should be doing but aren't. If you're skeptical about sidestepping all the criticism, ask when the last time beating yourself up accomplished anything good. For one, feeling guilty isn't particularly helpful. Giving yourself a hard time for not exercising, for example, rarely results in a workout. More often, negative self-talk is followed by a heavy sigh and a trip to the fridge for some Häagen Dazs. A phrase that acknowledges your desire, while not beating you up in the process, can help—such as, "If I really wanted to, I would work out." Try replacing all of your *shoulds* with, "If I really wanted to, I would..." and then notice how you feel.

Tricks of the Trade

A few tools of the trade can help you side-step stumbling blocks to healthy thinking. One of the foremost impediments, ripping the reigns right out from the best of intentions, is the mental circus that develops when we try not to think about something. Right now, try not thinking about a purple horse. Like a loop that eventually leaves us where we started, the harder we try to put it out of our minds the more the purple horse shows up. Using the phrase, "There it is again," works great here. Casually noticing that the purple horse has appeared, without judgment this time, allows it to just go away. Ahhh, there it is again. Gently, almost effortlessly, and without drama, the purple horse fades away.

But what if you're sorry to see him go? What if our purple horse is a real problem that needs real attention? Then give it the time and attention it deserves. Write about it, talk about it, get advice, and ask questions. Then, when you've done what you can do for that day and there is nothing more for you to do but obsess, take a look at your watch and set aside a specific time to worry about it some more rather than let it overtake the present moment. Let's say you decide to think about the issue at hand for a half hour at 3:00 p.m. At every intrusive thought, gently remind yourself that you'll stew about it at three o'clock. Then as soon as the little hand is on the three, go at it and give it all you've got. Then set up your next time to worry, say 9:00 p.m. Now you've allowed room for problem solving—or obsessing—without letting it overwhelm the rest of your life. Most of the time you'll discover that you really don't want to spend the half hour, or even ten minutes, fretting about something you can't control. But if not, it hasn't clouded your day or your judgment.

Short-circuiting your best efforts may be other people with their ideas, opinions, and judgments. Letting other people and their problems take up residence in your head, rent free, results in lackluster living at best, and can make you miserable in the process. Reclaiming that space in your head may require a few evictions, but the side effects—or benefits—can be a reduction in anxiety and depression. For Ellen Dracos Lemming, featured in *More* magazine, the epiphany came one night when she was worrying about work. Her husband asked her what she was afraid of. "That's when I decided to stop being afraid—of failing, of disappointing, of being unpopular. I began to give myself permission to be who I am. What are they going to do? Scream? Yell?" Donna Sturgess, Vice President of Innovation for GlaxoSmithKline adds, "you hit a fork in the road, say 'enough!'—and you either become an agent of change where you are or move on." One woman said, "Do something about it, forget it or forgive it."[270]

The health dividends of adjusting your thinking can be broad. In chapter 2 I alluded to a pilot study for people suffering from IBS (irritable bowel syndrome) using a ten-week home-based program. For IBS sufferers, abdominal pain and discomfort can be a way of life. But when participants learned to track their thoughts and upgrade their thinking, symptoms diminished by 70 percent, compared to only 7.5 percent in the non-participating group.[271] This type of training is called cognitive behavioral therapy, or CBT. In CBT self-limiting beliefs are targeted and replaced with accurate and supportive thinking.

As you can see, it takes only a short time to experience results—even boosting immune cells. In a collaborative study at Yale and the University of Pennsylvania, an eight-week course in relaxation techniques and cognitive therapy resulted in a sharp increase in the activity of natural killer cells.[272] You may recall that other studies have demonstrated that an apathetic attitude, lack of social support, and a passive coping style are linked to a reduction in these specialized immune cells.

In any given moment you have two powerful agents of change: your breath and your thoughts. CBT has been shown to be effective in treating depression as well. (Seeing a therapist specifically trained in this technique can speed progress or you can use the superb self-help tools in the Resource Guide; of course, if your depression is severe or life-threatening, professional help is highly advised.)

Ice Rocks

If our self-talk is about what we *don't* want, then like it or not, that's where we're headed. This was made rather obvious to me one blustery day skiing in the Alps. I was at the top of a steep slope, part of a several mile ski run into the Tyrolean village below. Now, I'm an okay skier. Not great, not awful, just okay. But I must have seemed nervous because the man next to me pointed out some large ice rocks to be wary of. They were huge. I determined to absolutely avoid those things. Keeping my eye firmly on the rocks, making sure to navigate around them, I got closer... and closer...there they are...as I plowed right into them, skis flying.

Later, after collecting my gear and picking my way down the mountain, other skiers kept asking if I was okay. I had taken my time brushing off the evidence (snow stuck everywhere) so I was a little miffed until I realized my forehead was cut and there was blood on my face. It was more like mud on my face—more embarrassed than injured.

What I learned was this: our skis, like our life, point in the direction we're looking. Make sure it's a direction you want to go. Focusing on our faults and our flaws may actually bring us more of what we *don't* want. By focusing on what we do want more of, maybe more compassion, tolerance, or peace, we'll be moving in the direction of our goals.

The Three Questions

Whatever our circumstances, these three questions can help unravel crooked thinking and keep us on target:

1. Is this line of thinking how I want to create my future?
2. Is it productive? Is it true?
3. Is it helping me now?

Let's take a quick look at each of these. *Number One: Is this line of thinking how I want to create my future?* We move in the direction we're facing. Unless we're problem solving or creating change, what we're looking at, focusing on, and thinking about creates our next moments. Remember the ice rocks. Enough said.

Number Two: Is it productive? Is it true? Mark Twain said a cat won't jump on a hot stove twice but he won't jump on a cold one either. Like the experienced cat, we can collect and collate the happenings of our life into a belief system that may not hold up if scrutinized. We want to actively challenge self-limiting beliefs and cultivate wonder and joy. But what if it is true and we don't like it? That's where Number Three comes in.

Number Three: Is this helping me now? Asking this question gives us a window of opportunity to shift our perception, freeing us from the confines of helplessness and the limitations of powerlessness. Railing against what is won't help. We escape the victim mentality if we take responsibility for the way we see the world and stop blaming others. At Harvard's Mind-Body Medicine training, a segment of the program refers to principles of CBT. A trick to rapidly reframe or adjust your thinking is: Stop. Breathe. Reflect and Choose. Whatever the situation, our thinking reveals the direction we're headed.

When healing, a strong sense of goodwill toward the self is essential. Most participants in the six-week class can readily quote, "Love thy neighbor," yet neglect the importance of the remainder, "as thyself." How well can we love another if we are stingy, harsh, and critical with ourselves? We're often willing to do for others what we aren't willing to do for ourselves. Caretaking—taking care of others without self-nurturing—is like being a gourmet chef and not eating. No matter how great your cooking, you will still starve to death.

One of my group participants brought in a story to illustrate the importance of this truth from the book *Chicken Soup for the Soul*, entitled "All the Good Things," by Helen P. Mrosla.[273] Helen was teaching what was called "new math" and the students were anxious, irritable, and disruptive with her and with each other. So she had the students write the nicest things they could say about each other and hand in their papers to her. Helen writes:

> That Saturday, I wrote down the name of each student on a separate sheet of paper, and I listed what everyone else had said about that individual. On Monday I gave each student his or her list. Before long, the entire class was smiling. "Really?" I heard whispered. "I never knew that meant anything to anyone!" "I didn't know others liked me so much!" No one ever mentioned those papers in class again. I never knew if they discussed them after class or with

their parents, but it did not matter. The exercise had accomplished its purpose. The students were happy with themselves and one another again. That group of students moved on.

[Helen continues.] Several years later, after I returned from vacation, my parents met me at the airport…'The Eklunds called last night,' [my father] began. 'Really?' I said. 'I haven't heard from them in years. I wonder how Mark is.' Dad responded quietly, 'Mark was killed in Vietnam,' he said. 'The funeral is tomorrow, and his parents would like it if you could attend.'

…After the funeral, most of Mark's former classmates headed to Chuck's [a classmate] farmhouse for lunch. Mark's mother and father were there, obviously waiting for me. 'We want to show you something,' his father said, taking a wallet out of his pocket. 'They found this on Mark when he was killed. We thought you might recognize it.' Opening the billfold, he carefully removed two worn pieces of notebook paper that had obviously been taped, folded, and refolded many times. I knew without looking that the papers were the ones on which I had listed all the good things each of Mark's classmates had said about him. 'Thank you so much for doing that,' Mark's mother said. 'As you can see, Mark treasured it.'

Mark's classmates started to gather around us. Charlie smiled rather sheepishly and said, 'I still have my list. It's in the top drawer of my desk at home.' Chuck's wife said, 'Chuck asked me to put his in our wedding album.' 'I have mine too,' Marilyn said. 'It's in my diary.' Then Vicki, another classmate, reached into her pocketbook, took out her wallet and showed her worn and frazzled list to the group. 'I carry this with me at all times,' Vicki said without batting an eyelash. 'I think we all saved our lists.'

We may not have had such a teacher, but how do we respond to the sweet words or kindnesses we do receive? At a conference I attended, the presenter used a cylinder, a funnel, and pitcher of water to show

how many of us receive praise. Turning the funnel upside down she pours water into the funnel's tiny spout. Only a small amount of water actually gets into the container; the rest splashes outside the funnel and cylinder, missing the mark completely. She likened the cylinder to our brain: when we reject or ignore compliments, very little gets inside. The students in Helen's class had their funnels set to receive; we can too, by remembering and reflecting with gratitude upon the warm words we receive from others.

The Third C: Challenge

The Three Questions and the three Cs keep us on track. In chapter 8 you examined two of those, Commitment and Control—action qualities, but the Third C, Challenge, is about how we view what we can't control or change. When I first met Joan, it was hard to imagine that anything could possibly be wrong. Beautiful, smart, and successful, she was pregnant with her second child. But five months into the pregnancy, her doctors discovered advanced colon cancer. In all the medical literature worldwide, there were only three cases like hers. Without chemotherapy she would be unlikely to live long enough to deliver the baby. With chemotherapy, the specialist told Joan she could expect multiple congenital defects. For these reasons doctors advised her to abort. But Joan believed that the baby saved her life, that if she hadn't been pregnant, the cancer would have gone undetected. Joan's specialists disagreed with her decision to keep the baby, but supported her right to choose for herself, and adjusted the chemotherapy to a slightly lower dose. On the one hand, Joan felt morally relieved. On the other, the decision left her alone without a single other case in medical literature she could rely on for comfort or hope. In tandem with all of this—if you can imagine—Joan's ten-year-old son

Life is seldom as unendurable as, to judge by the facts, it ought to be.

—BROOKS ATKINSON

had just been diagnosed with osteosarcoma—a type of bone cancer—the previous year.

Was she terrified? Absolutely. But to face the months ahead, Joan needed to listen to her heart and deal with her own fears, while allowing hope for the unexpected to take root. For Joan, this meant soothing and calming herself, creating an environment that was nourishing, and releasing the limiting paradigm set before her. Joan heard about the six-week class our cancer center offered, and even though she lived in North Carolina she made the trip to attend each week. As her days were relegated to driving to doctor appointments for herself and her son, she made a habit of deep breathing (for two minutes she told me) every time she touched her car keys. When she learned about imagery, Joan imagined a protective barrier shielding her baby from the toxic effects of chemotherapy. In her mind's eye she also targeted the treatment toward all the cancer cells, and away from the healthy ones. At the end of every imagery session, she would see herself hardy and strong, delivering a healthy baby. Four months later that is exactly what she did. Her daughter is over three years old now, beautiful in every way, and Joan remains cancer-free. And her son continues to be in remission.

Predictions. Prognosis. Statistical outcomes. What looked like reality for Joan was nothing of the sort. She could have spent those months in anxious misery, and certainly there were many times when she was concerned and worried. But she refused to allow the unknown to mar either the joy she felt each day, or the feeling that in this moment, until she absolutely knew otherwise, all was well. We know not every case has an ending like this one, which reminds me of a Chinese proverb: he who imagines bad things happening, experiences them twice. Once we've done the best we can do, there's no need to remain in expectation of the worst—it may arrive or it may not.

Having the courage to recognize when or how our current frame of reference is edging us in, is the first step in being able to create a new meaning that will support and empower our purpose. You might have seen this popular brainteaser before. I first saw it in *Minding the Body, Mending the Mind,* where Joan Borysenko uses it as an apt example of reframing.

Get Started Now: Getting Out of Our Box

Here are the rules:

Connect all nine dots using four, straight, continuous lines, no curves allowed.

Your pencil must stay on the paper.

In other words, you can't lift it up and make disconnected lines. Hint: You have to get out of the box first!

See the next page for the solution.

Anne had raised her children and taken care of her husband, and just as she was beginning to relish the possibilities for herself she was diagnosed with multiple myeloma (MM), a blood cancer. Crushed with fear and disappointment, she determined to view the diagnosis as a challenge to be met. In an exercise designed to elicit meaning from illness, she wrote this poem:

Turnabout is fair play. Tell the Cancer that—Watch it squirm like I squirmed. Stop it cold—in its tracks—whatever cliché works. Make

it know that anything it can do, I can do—with more verve, more
gusto, more determination than cancer ever could muster. I won't
turn away from the battle—I hate to lose. I'll keep turning up the
heat—Until I finally emerge the winner in a mortal combat I never
sought but will not turn from.

Anne continued to view her situation as a challenge, avidly pursuing her doctorate in literature and completing her dissertation, while
dealing with broken bones (from the MM) and pneumonia, switching
from one chemotherapeutic protocol to another, and mourning the per-
manent loss of sensation in her legs and feet. For Anne to adopt this attitude, she had to develop a frame of reference that promoted her sense
of personal power. In choosing to envision the challenge she faced as a
battle between herself and the cancer, a new meaning was born, one that
allowed her to pursue her dreams while she could. The poem she wrote
above was inscribed on the back of her funeral announcement when she
passed away a few years later.

Get Started Now: Getting Out of Our Box

Solution:

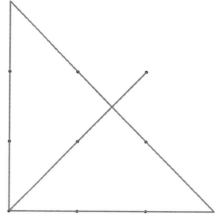

To solve this puzzle, we have to get out of the box. Attempting to connect the
dots while confining ourselves mentally to the linear lines of a square is impos-

sible. But once we can see that the square is self-imposed, we can move beyond it. And so it is in life. As soon as we identify alternate choices and options—whether or not we like them—we're out of the box! Anything that gets us out of the box expands our perception and offers us more opportunities.

One of the most creative cases of reframing I have come across lately is from a woman in our group, Carol, who has lymphoma. She is thirty-nine years old and has four children under the age of ten, a part time job as a librarian, a loving husband, and a nasty mother-in-law. Fortunately for Carol her mother-in-law's visits are rare, but when they happen Carol feels resentful and depressed. Her counselor made excellent suggestions, but for Carol it was a lunchtime discussion with three girlfriends who had mother-in-law issues of their own that really made the difference, when they artfully reframed their situation by forming a club. Meeting each month, the mean mother-in-law club was based on points. The more horrible the story, the more points. Whoever wound up with the most points would be treated to lunch. The next visit, Carol was practically gleeful with her mother-in-law's caustic criticism. Oooh, that's a good one, she would think. Sometimes there would be so many she would have to rip out her journal to catch the flow. Carol told our group that she had started to actually look forward to her visits because she knew the free lunch was hers.

While no one is advocating putting up with verbal abuse or chronic criticism, sharing the stories of your life with supportive friends or being a part of a group can help us see an opportunity or a chance for things to be different and offers a rich reference for getting out of the box. The skills you learned in chapters 2 and 4 (diaphragmatic breathing along with relaxation and imagery) lend a hand, too. In a more relaxed frame of mind, new associations and potential solutions are more easily made while we virtually reprogram our standard response to stressors or problems. Cultivating awareness helps us to move beyond a narrow worldview by identifying the choices we have. Someone once told me (I don't remember whom) that there are three types of people in the world: those who are angry about the past, fearful about the future, or excited about the here and now.

The following Chinese fable looks at this from a different angle. Unforeseen occurrences—wrong place, wrong time, or right place, right time—happen to all of us. Making too much of either gets in the way of appreciating the present. Dr. Brehony shares the tale: The farmer's horse runs away into the mountains. "Bad luck," the neighbor says. "Good luck, bad luck, who knows," says the farmer. The next day the runaway horse returns, followed by six wild horses. They race into the corral and the farmer locks the gate. "What good luck," the neighbor says. "Good luck, bad luck, who knows?" says the farmer. The next day the farmer's son, trying to break one of the wild horses, falls off and breaks his leg. "What bad luck," the neighbor says. "Good luck, bad luck, who knows?" says the farmer. The very next day the army comes by conscripting all able-bodied young men for a bloody foreign war. The farmer's son can't go, of course—he's got a broken leg. "What good luck," the neighbor says. "Good luck, bad luck, who knows?" says the farmer. Labels such as "bad luck," or "good luck," can block our ability to move beyond the particulars and find a larger meaning or perspective. The final chapter takes us to the heart of the matter.

Meaning: The Heart of the Matter

Fate leads the willing, and drags along the reluctant.
—LUCIUS ANNAEUS SENECA,
FIRST CENTURY PHILOSOPHER

They met in medical school and married during residency. As a couple they carefully calculated their options and opportunities—where to live and where to work—planning their lives with precision and care. When their daughter, Elizabeth, was born, they were prepared; everything was in perfect order and stayed that way for a few years. Then, during a routine blood test, their four-year-old little girl was diagnosed with leukemia. With a medical treatment plan firmly in place, the parents prioritized their daughter's needs, especially her emotional ones.

Concerned about the effect Elizabeth's hair loss would have and worried about teasing from playmates, the parents purchased every possible wig and jazzy head covering before she lost a single hair. Not breathing a word of what was ahead, their plan was to have the fun pieces ready to go at the first sign of tears.

But there weren't any. After chemo, Elizabeth's head got itchy and she started pulling at her hair. It was loose and didn't take much, but the more she scratched and pulled, the faster it came out and there she was, beautifully bald. Declining any covering, her mother saw Elizabeth's friends making faces and pointing at her. "What happened to your hair?" "It was itchy so I pulled it out." And that was that. The playmates shrugged, as if it made perfect sense to them and they all went back to their game.

The meaning behind the hair loss was different for Elizabeth than it was for her parents. Our meaning is defined in part by our perspective. For Elizabeth, it was itchy and uncomfortable and so she had no hair. For her parents, the hair loss represented the serious challenge she faced. The implications, though, lie beyond perspective, filtering down into our cells, in between the microscopic crevices of dendrites and synapses, trickling into channels of communication that determine a physical reaction, even affecting how we feel and respond to pain.

The Anzio Effect

The Anzio effect is just one example of such a thing—the by-product of perspective.[274] A busy fishing port and tourist destination, Anzio lies about thirty miles south of Rome. Known as Antium in ancient times and frequented by emperors, the town still has the remains of villas dotting the shoreline. But in an amphibious landing by the Allies on January 22, 1944, Anzio became home to a four-month battle that would overtake the seaside town, leaving it laden with casualties. Over sixty thousand civilians and soldiers overwhelmed the hospitals and medical care centers.

In this setting, Harvard anesthesiologist Henry Beecher found that only 32 percent of soldiers undergoing surgery for serious wounds rated their pain as "significant," as opposed to 83 percent of civilians who faced the same surgery back at Massachusetts General Hospital. Professor of Neuroscience at California State University Steve Suter, Ph.D., explains Beecher's belief that the level of pain had everything to do with the meaning ascribed to the event. In this case, civilians viewed the surgery itself as life-threatening; the soldiers, on the other hand, had barely escaped with their lives from a perilous combat zone and were overcome with relief and thankfulness.

In a recent communication Dr. Suter wrote that it's not a big leap to extend this to coping with illness in general. We do not have total control over what happens to us, only how we respond—which has a lot to do with how we interpret the events of our lives. The following are five ways we can interpret illness depending on the meaning we assign to it:

1. a challenge to be met
2. a form of punishment
3. an opportunity for personal growth
4. an event signifying irreparable loss or damage to ourselves
5. a welcome escape from responsibilities

(For years I credited Dr. Suter with this excellent recap, but he declines the credit—and neither he nor I know who to give it to here, but it's too smart to leave out!)

We need expanded vision to cope with the complexities of life in general, but especially when our sense of meaning is challenged by catastrophic events and suffering. At times like these our meaning needs to be reclaimed, or refreshed. It no longer surprises me when patients associate their disease with an emotional cause or loss of meaning, but at first this startled me. Here I was introducing mind-body medicine to people who had never heard of such a thing and were unfamiliar with the science. Yet without prompting, often in their introductory comments to the group, references to loss, trauma, or grief would inevitably be linked to the diagnosis. At Harvard's mind-body programs participants draw a timeline connecting the significant events of their lives with corresponding emotional and physical states. In a training program for health professionals, Dr. Webster brought in several timelines patients had completed—gorgeous poster-sized works of art. You don't have to do anything quite so elaborate (unless you choose to do so), but you can scribble a timeline in your journal or use crayons and markers to make more of a splash.

Get Started Now: Your Personal Timeline

Significant people. Inspirational moments. The birth of a child. All of these have left an indelible imprint on your life. Reflect on your life in a linear way, and draw a timeline or a rough sketch of your life so far. If you are sixty, you may decide to divide up your timeline into twelve five-year segments. Then fill in special people, remarkable events, job changes, relocations, or the loss of someone dear. You've already seen how helpful it can be to find a deeper meaning in a challenge or a setback. Note how resilient or courageous you've been over the years! See if you can determine how you've grown and changed as a result of all of these things, both "good" and "bad." Look up at the five ways we respond to illness. Based on your past experience, what might help you with any current challenge you are facing? Is there a broader meaning you can bring to the table? Play with it over a few days and see what comes up for you.

No one is saying that loss of meaning or stressful events are the sole cause of our health problems. But we have choices in how we view our world, and how we view change itself. Connecting the dots on our timeline can help us reevaluate the meaning or importance we have attached to certain events and help us reestablish a frame of reference that is constructive or supportive. This enhanced vantage point can reconnect us with our purpose or redefine it. During the Holocaust, clinical psychologist Viktor Frankl chronicled the collective search for meaning in the face of unspeakable crimes. As hate's ravenous appetite consumed his practice, his home, and the lives of his entire family with the exception of his sister Stella, Frankl began to survey the nightmare around him. Imprisoned in four different concentration camps, including the most infamous, Auschwitz, he was able to observe firsthand the link between self-worth and the ability to survive.

Frankl discerned that individuals who could find a larger meaning in their suffering were often able to withstand the cruelty, deprivation, and disease of the camps. Armored with an unquenchable zeal for life, and in tandem with their quest for meaning, they made a personal decision not to relinquish themselves to the hate that threatened their survival. Documenting what attitude could do long before we could isolate its chemical components, Frankl writes, "We must never forget that we may also find meaning in life even when confronted with a hopeless situation, when facing a fate that cannot be changed. For what then matters is to bear witness to the uniquely human potential at its best, which is to transform a personal tragedy into a triumph, to turn one's predicament into a human achievement."[275] His book *Man's Search for Meaning* has sold over nine million copies worldwide. The Library of Congress has declared it to be among the top ten most influential books of all time.

Joining that distinctive nomination will likely be award-winning author Kathleen Brehony's comprehensive work *After the Darkest Hour: How Suffering Begins the Journey to Wisdom,*[276] a guide to reclaiming meaning and reigniting our lives with passion and grace. It is human nature to want to fast forward through the painful and difficult parts of our lives. When diagnosed with serious illness, we may find it appealing to focus entirely on our treatment options, hoping to turn the corner as rapidly as possible.

In doing so, we risk losing a valuable opportunity. There is no greater motivator for personal growth or change than that of a catastrophic illness. We can be well developed in some aspects, perhaps in a role as a professional or as a parent, but other facets of our character may not have the same luster. Coping with chronic illness, perhaps in situations where we are no longer able to function in our usual capacity, provides a unique platform upon which to explore other aspects of our self. It can be an opportunity to flesh out, define, and polish the rest of our potential qualities. Because to truly live consciously and mindfully—to find hope in the deepest sense—means that we live fully regardless of outcomes, blood results, and other diagnostic aids.

When I lost nearly all of my blood in a medical accident and the doctors didn't know why, I was astonished to discover how results-oriented I became. I graphed each small movement of my red blood cells from my hospital bed. When they reached 4.7, I cheered. The next day when they were 4.5, I despaired. After days of this sort of thing and no end in sight, my father entered my hospital room clutching a well-worn copy of Rudyard Kipling's poem, "If." I wondered what was up. What about this particular poem could possibly help me now? I braced myself for platitudes and the plug for positive thinking that was surely coming. He began, "If you can dream—and not make dreams your master; If you can think—and not make thoughts your aim; [but it was the following line he was after] If you can meet with triumph and disaster; And treat those two imposters just the same..." Of course. That was supposed to be my line, wasn't it? Treating outcomes like the imposters they are.

Amidst all the scientific research of mind-body communication systems and issues of personal responsibility, there remains the humbling and awesome task faced by each individual—how to live with uncertainty. One woman described her diagnosis this way: "A door slams in your face. Suddenly you're in a parallel universe doing the same things as everyone else but you're not the same and you never will be." But that threat—the life-changing diagnosis—can be a gift, and one of permission to savor the moment. When we come face-to-face with our own mortality, priorities rapidly change. We want more satisfaction in our lives and we begin to search for it. We are shortchanged when we focus so intently on beating the disease that we lose sight of what makes living worthwhile and meaningful, because eventually, everyone dies. Facing our own mortality demands the ultimate act of creativity: designing a life that suits us.

Cancer is a serious crisis—but isn't life a matter of adapting to one change after another? I believe we must continually adapt to survive, and as life goes on, we can thrive on living. There's no reason we cannot maintain a fine quality of life during a life-threatening crisis. The diagnosis of cancer is not an automatic death warrant that demands that the patient and his family stop living.

—Carl Simonton, M.D.

Doing that demands finding joy apart from diagnostics and test results. From the time she was nineteen years old, cysts had to be drained regularly from Leah's breasts. When she was in her forties, both Leah's sister and aunt had died from breast cancer and her mother had been diagnosed. Leah had mammograms every six months, but dense breast tissue made reading the results difficult, and between mammograms she was found to have metastatic stage-four breast cancer. It had invaded her bones, and there were spots on her skull, in her leg, and eroding her hip. A special surgical procedure placed pins in both of her hips, and a double mastectomy was followed by high dose chemotherapy.

Leah and her husband reevaluated their life. Although her prognosis was dire, for the next four years while she was on chemotherapy, they traveled, met their goals, and lived mindfully, striving not to base their feelings on test results or outcomes. When the treatment had done what it could do, and it was clear that Leah was dying, hospice provided comfort and care. When the doctors told her that she had perhaps only a day or two left to live, her husband gathered their children and family so she could say goodbye. Leah had known the moment was coming and she was prepared. But time passed. Two days, then three. A week. Her husband decided to bring Leah home, so she could die there. Unable to eat or drink and without an IV line, her husband used an eyedropper to deliver small amounts of nutritious fluids to keep her more comfortable. Weeks passed.

For reasons that no one can explain, Leah improved. Gradually, the cancer regressed, but not to the point where she was truly cancer-free. Still, they had a reprieve. Not taking anything for granted, Leah followed scrupulous nutritional guidelines and took great care of her health. Because of side effects from chemotherapy, Leah didn't immediately respond when digestive troubles began. But when her symptoms intensified, a scope revealed gastrointestinal cancer (not metastasized breast cancer—this was a new type of cancer altogether). She went in for surgery so they could remove her stomach, but when they opened her up the cancer was too far advanced. They sewed up the incision, and once again told her she didn't have long to live. Yet Leah rallied; it would be more than another year before she would die. She and her husband never denied the reality, but refused to base their attitude on test results or outcomes, filling the precious years they found together with purpose and joy.

The awareness that death is not a failure—we are all terminal—allows us to experience a unique type of freedom. In the face of death, excuses and rationalizations for denying ourselves a full and rich life fall away, for what else is there to lose? Facing our own mortality allows us to appreciate the present, live in the moment, and create a new way of being. Designing a life that suits us, that stimulates us, one that makes us feel vibrantly and passionately alive, may be our greatest work.

After one Saturday too many of forfeiting playing with my stepchildren to work on this manuscript, they began to complain. Loudly. "When is that thing going to be finished?!" "For all the time you're spending, it had better hit the *New York Times* best seller list!" "This is taking forever. Don't you have a deadline or something?" Amid promises that it was almost finished, thirteen-year-old Thomas let slip that the title of my book, "didn't really do it" for him. So I asked him what he had in mind. Since everyone had forgotten what it was about, they asked for a recap. After a brief pause he said, "I think this says it better:

Stop Living Like You're Already Dead: The Inspiring 6-Week Program That Helps You Liven Up." We were all laughing, but he's got the idea, doesn't he?

The war on disease will rage on and move forward, from research laboratories and epidemiological studies, to specialty and primary medical practices, to the alternative and holistic community. Rallying our resources to heal from within, though, gives us a measure of insight and personal grace. Though a remission from disease is not our primary goal, a by-product of living life in this fashion can indeed be beating the odds. As you have seen, belief in and commitment to self mobilizes our will to live and thereby our immune system. This is powerful medicine. It is also mysterious and raises far more questions than we have answers for. Skeptics counter that until we have all the answers, there's no need to make programs like this an adjunct to medical care. Neuroscientist David Felten, M.D., Ph.D., and director of the Center for Neuroimmunology at the Loma Linda University School of Medicine, responds to the call for definitive answers in his essay found in the classic text *Psychoneuroimmunology*. I first read his heart-stopping commentary in Dreher's book *Mind-Body Unity*, and am honored to have permission to share it with you:

> Although it is tempting for the basic scientist to ignore or deny that which cannot be explained on a mechanistic level, I am one such basic scientist who has been touched by the example of my mother, Jane Felten, a courageous woman who faced life crippled with polio and beset with medical problems, but whose determination and irrepressible spirit seemed to carry her through almost unbelievable medical adversity. Paralyzed at 8 years of age, she faced more than 10 orthopedic procedures to fuse bones of the lower extremities to allow her to stand with crutches. She never thought anyone would want to marry her, but she found a kind, gracious, and loving man, Harold Felten, whose example has been an inspiration to all who

know him. She was told repeatedly by the medical establishment never to risk having children or trying to raise them but managed to have two sons at some risk to her own well-being. She spent many long and frustrating years learning to balance on crutches while gripping the tops with just her upper arms, to permit some use of her hands to care for her children, despite the inevitable damage to the brachial plexus this caused. Never once did I hear her complain about her affliction or her lot in life; rather, she took joy in her husband and children, her faith, and the kindness of others. She faced repeated cardiac problems with the attitude that it was a small price to pay for the good life she had been permitted. She faced repeated bouts of pneumonia and pulmonary problems with an astonishing determination to fight back and recover, which she managed to do for many years, beyond anyone's expectations. And when she faced ultimate deterioration, mental confusion, and death, in her more lucid moments she expressed gratitude to those who showed care and kindness to her.

Do we know the extent to which Jane Felten was able to assist herself to recover from illness and fight back from adversity, through some of the interactions described in this book? No. Do we understand how the support of a loving and caring husband contributed to neural signaling that helped her through overwhelming adversity, such as repeated bouts of pneumonia and cardiac failure? No. But does that mean that such factors are irrelevant just because we do not yet understand the mechanisms that underlie them? And does this mean that the example of Jane Felten and many others like her should be put aside, to be dismissed as mere anecdote or mythology? I think not. Rather, her example should serve as a constant reminder that healing involves far more than pharmacological mechanisms, and that the physician's role includes more than just the manipulation of currently understood physiological mechanisms. And her example should serve as an inspiration for us to explore further the scientific foundations and to unravel the mechanisms of interaction of brain, behavior, and immunity, so that in the future we will understand better how attitude, will, stressors, and positive emotions are expressed in the periphery, including the immune system.[277]

Jane Felten beat the odds. Yet even with such a tremendous outcome, we are really not talking here about a "cure," but as Dee Brigham said, a dimension of spirit and a sense of inner power. This shift in focus can be invigorating. There is great joy and freedom to be had in this so-called paradox, that to live fully and meaningfully one must accept the reality of one's death. Yet, in doing so, our orientation toward life shifts. What was once significant now becomes simply mundane—new priorities and pleasures surface. The meaning and significance varies; it's the process of discovery that makes each journey unique.

The concept is neatly summarized by a woman who wrote me, "When you can't think big anymore, you think small. And then everything's important...and you don't want to miss a thing. Everything is precious." Dick Haddow, a 6'4" Scotsman with tremendous vital energy and a wicked sense of humor, described a pivotal moment after dealing with serious illness for five years. Working hard outdoors one day, he saw a butterfly; duly noting it, he resumed work and then paused. He asked himself how he would feel and what he would do if this were his last day on earth. Putting down his tools, he paused to enjoy this sublime gift of creation.

We do not have to wait until we have a life-threatening or chronic illness to develop an enhanced way of relating to the world. We can apply the principles of healing to every aspect of our lives and to a variety of new, unexpected situations, and experience a more congruent way of living, a more harmonious way of being in our own body. In doing so, we will make room for miracles in our lives—for sixty days, or sixty years—however long we may live.

RESOURCE GUIDE

For more information or to schedule a phone consultation with the author, please see her website at www.brendastockdale.com.

Chapter One

They Can't Find Anything Wrong, David Clarke, M.D.

The Inflammation Cure, William Meggs, M.D.

YOU: The Owner's Manual: An Insider's Guide to the Body that Will Make You Healthier and Younger, Memmet Oz, M.D.

Chapter Two

Spontaneous Remission database at the Institute of Noetic Sciences: www.noetic.org/research/sr/biblio.html.

Newsletters:

On adrenal fatigue and stress: www.womentowomen.com.

Susan Lark, M.D., newsletter: www.drlark.com.

Cardiologist Stephen Sinatra, M.D., newsletter: www.drsinatra.com.

Books:

Mind-Body Unity: A New Vision for Mind-Body Science and Medicine, Henry Dreher, M.A.

Change Your Beliefs, Change Your Life, Nicholas Hall, Ph.D.

Cancer as a Turning Point, Lawrence LeShan, Ph.D.

The Biology of Belief, Bruce Lipton, Ph.D.

When the Body Says No, Gabor Mate, M.D.

Molecules of Emotion, Candace Pert, Ph.D.

The Psychobiology of Gene Expression, Ernest Rossi, Ph.D.

Mind Over Back Pain, John Sarno, M.D.

Consultations:

Medical research and cancer guides consultations, contact Henry Dreher at: 212. 228. 0322 or www.henrydreher.com.

Ralph Moss, Ph.D., is a science writer and medical investigator specializing in cancer: www.cancerdecisions.com.

Chapter Three

Temperature bulbs: handheld temperature bulbs (BF-199) can be ordered from Echo, Inc. at 937-322-4972.

Biodots and other tools: www.stressmarket.com.

Adrenal/cortisol testing: www.diagnostechs.com.

Andrew Weil, M.D., offers CDs and other information on healthy breathing. For more, go to: www.drweil.com.

The Resperate device uses paced guided breathing exercises with headphones that can help with blood pressure: www.resperate.com.

StressEraser monitors your heart rate variability and helps with breathing: www.stresseraser.com.

Great site on healthy breathing: saveyourself.ca/articles/respiration-connection.php.

Books:

The Slow Down Diet, Marc David.

The Relaxation and Stress Reduction Workbook, sixth edition, Martha Davis et al.

The Healthy Mind Healthy Body Handbook, David Sobel, M.D., and Robert Ornstein, Ph.D.

Secrets of Optimal Natural Breathing, M.G. White.

Chapter Four

Health programs and training centers:

Commonweal offers a variety of programs: www.commonweal.org/programs.

For retreats, books, and tapes, Exceptional Cancer Patients. Barry Bittman, M.D., Meadville Medical Center: 814-337-8192 or www.mind-body.org.

Harvard's Eight Day Programs: The Mind/Body Medical Institute at Harvard University: 617-632-9530, or www.mindbody.harvard.edu.

Center for Mind-Body Medicine, directed by James Gordon, M.D.: 202-966-7338 or www.cmbm.org.

Lawrence LeShan's Five Day Programs: ww.cancerasaturningpoint.org/fiveday.htm.

Simonton Cancer Center: offers a five day educational and psychotherapeutic program for cancer patients and their spouses. 310-459-4434.

Books:

Staying Well With Guided Imagery, Belleruth Naparstek, M.S.W. Check out recent studies using imagery and relaxation techniques on her website at www.healthjourneys.com. Click on "Hot Research" and use the pull-down menu to access a variety of health conditions.

Invisible Heroes: Survivors of Trauma and How They Heal, Belleruth Naparstek, M.S.W.

An excellent guide for clinicians: Imagery for Getting Well, Deirdre Brigham, M.A., L.M.F.T., M.P.H.

Healing Yourself, Martin Rossman, M.D.

Guided Imagery for Self-Healing, Martin Rossman, M.D.

Fighting Cancer from Within: How to Use the Power of Your Mind for Healing, Martin Rossman, M.D.

CDs:

For a catalogue of CDs, videos, and books, see www.healthjourneys.com.

For books and relaxation CDs, The Mind/Body Medical Institute at Harvard University: 617-632-9530 or www.mindbody.harvard.edu.

Beree Darby, Ph.D., offers health and performance enhancement CDs at: 352-375-4441 or www.drdarby.com.

Emmett Miller, M.D., offers Healing Journey for general wellness, Positive Imagery for People with Cancer, and if you have back pain, insomnia, or high blood pressure he offers CDs for these as well: 800-52-TAPES or www.drmiller.com.

Imagery for surgery:

Emmett Miller, M.D.: "Successful Surgery and Recovery" can be found at: www.drmiller.com.

For relaxation tapes and the PIP Surgical Audiotape Series by Linda Rodgers: 914-232-6405.

Martin Rossman, M.D.: "Preparing for Surgery" and "Relax into Healing" can be found at www.thehealingmind.org/index.php/more/surgery/. His website also includes recent studies and investigations.

For referrals to guided imagery therapists contact The Academy for Guided Imagery at: 800-726-2070.

Chapter Five

Exceptional Cancer Patients, ECaP, Medical Director: Barry Bittman, M.D.: 814-337-8192 or www.mind-body.org.

Hemi-Sync has a variety of psychoacoustic CDs: www.hemi-sync.com.

Kelly Howell also offers psychoacoustic CDs including Mind/Body Healing at www.brainsync.com.

The American Music Therapy Association: 301-589-3300.

Rhythmic Medicine—Music with a Purpose: 913-696-1990 for information.

The Tomatis Method. Sound Listening and Learning Center, Tomatis USA, Phoenix, Arizona 85016: 602-381-0086. Tomatis International, Paris, France: 01-53-53-42-40. The Listening Centre, Tomatis Canada, Toronto, Ontario: 416-588-4136.

Andrew Weil, Sound Mind, Sound Body: Music for Healing (CD).

Books:

The Mozart Effect: Tapping the Power of Music to Heal the Body, Strengthen the Mind, and Unlock the Creative Spirit, Don Campbell.

Chapter Six

Keirsey: www.keirsey.com or see his book Please Understand Me, second edition.

Books:

Head First: The Biology of Hope and the Healing Power of the Human Spirit, Norman Cousins.

Finding Flow: The Psychology of Engagement with Everyday Life, Mihaly Csikszentmihalyi, Ph.D.

QED: The Strange Theory of Light and Matter, Richard Feynman, Ph.D.

The Journey Through Cancer: Healing & Transforming the Whole Person, Jeremy Geffen, M.D.

Focusing, Eugene Gendling, Ph.D.

For a list of affirmations based on illness or symptoms see the book *Heal Your Body*, Louise Hay.

Beyond Technique: Psychotherapy for the 21st Century, Lawrence LeShan, Ph.D.

Deep Healing, Emmett Miller, M.D.

Happiness Is a Serious Problem: A Human Nature Repair Manual, Dennis Prager, Ph.D.

Kitchen Table Wisdom, Rachel Naomi Remen, M.D.

Chapter Seven

Adverse Childhood Experience Study (ACE): www.cdc.gov/nccdphp/ACE/.

Dr. Pennebaker's state of the art computer generated feedback will take a look at your perceptions and the way you see yourself and your world. Try it at www.utpsyc.org.

For workshops in journal writing, Center for Journal Therapy: 888-421-2298 or www.journaltherapy.com.

For workshops on journal writing, Dialogue House Associates: 800-221-5844 or www.intensivejournal.org.

Books:

Making Peace with Your Past: The Six Essential Steps to Enjoy a Great Future, Harold Bloomfield, M.D.

When Your Heart Speaks, Take Good Notes: The Healing Power of Writing, Susan Borkin

The Artist's Way, Julia Cameron and Mark Bryan.

The Creative Journal: The Art of Finding Yourself, Lucia Cappacione, Ph.D.

Narrative Medicine: Honoring the Stories of Illness, Rita Charon, M.D.

Writing as a Way of Healing: How Telling Our Stories Transforms Our Lives, Louise DeSalvo.

The Secret World of Drawings, Greg Furth, Ph.D.

Second Opinion, Leath Kendrick (poems of a journey through cancer)

Writing for Your Life, Deena Metzger, M.A.

Invisible Heroes: Survivors of Trauma and How They Heal, Belleruth Naparstek, M.S.W.

Heartbreak and Heart Disease: A Mind/Body Prescription for Healing the Heart, Stephen Sinatra, M.D.

Moods and Feelings List

Abandoned	Antisocial	Bored
Accepted	Anxious	Brave
Acknowledged	Appreciated	Brittle
Affectionate	Appreciative	Broken
Afraid	Apprehensive	Bruised
Agitated	Ashamed	Burdened
Aggravated	Awed	Calm
Aggressive	Awkward	Capable
Alarmed	Belittled	Cheerful
Alienated	Betrayed	Defeated
Alone	Bewildered	Defective
Amazed	Bitter	Dejected
Amorous	Blah	Delighted
Amused	Blessed	Demoralized
Angry	Blocked	Depressed
Annoyed	Blue	Desolate

Despairing	Grateful	Mistreated
Desperate	Grumpy	Misunderstood
Despondent	Guilty	Morose
Disconnected	Happy	Needed
Discouraged	Hateful	Neglected
Disgraced	Healthy	Nervous
Disinterested	Helpless	Numb
Dissatisfied	Hopeful	Offended
Disturbed	Hopeless	Oppressed
Doubtful	Humiliated	Optimistic
Downcast	Hurt	Ostracized
Dreadful	Ignored	Outraged
Ecstatic	Impatient	Overwhelmed
Embarrassed	Impotent	Panicky
Empowered	Inadequate	Passionate
Encumbered	Incompetent	Playful
Energized	Ineffective	Pleased
Enraged	Inferior	Powerless
Enthusiastic	Insecure	Powerful
Envious	Insignificant	Pressured
Euphoric	Inspired	Proud
Excited	Intimidated	Puzzled
Excluded	Irritable	Regretful
Exhausted	Isolated	Rejected
Exhilarated	Jealous	Rejuvenated
Fantastic	Jittery	Relaxed
Fearful	Joyous	Relieved
Foolish	Jumpy	Resentful
Forgiven	Justified	Respected
Frantic	Lifeless	Restless
Free	Lonely	Ridiculed
Frightened	Lost	Ridiculous
Frustrated	Loved	Sad
Fulfilled	Loving	Safe
Furious	Marvelous	Satisfied
Glad	Miserable	Scared

Serene	Thrilled	Valued
Shaky	Triumphant	Vengeful
Shocked	Trusting	Vindicated
Skeptical	Unappreciated	Victimized
Slighted	Uncertain	Victorious
Sorry	Uncomfortable	Vulnerable
Stifled	Understood	Wanted
Stuck	Uneasy	Welcomed
Spiteful	Unhappy	Well
Supported	Unimportant	Whole
Surprised	Unloved	Wonderful
Suspicious	Unstable	Wounded
Terrified	Unsure	Worried
Thankful	Upset	Worthless
Threatened	Uptight	Worthy

Chapter Eight

American Association for Therapeutic Humor, www.AATH.org.

Loretta LaRoche's CDs, *Relax, You May Only Have a Few Minutes Left* and *The Humor Potential*. At 800-998-2324 or www.lorettalaroche.com.

Dr. Al Siebert's Resiliency Quiz at www.resiliencycenter.com.

Adrenal/cortisol testing: www.diagnostechs.com.

For research on Juice Plus, www.juiceplus.com/research.

Center for Mind-Body Medicine, www.cmbm.org.

For information on functional medicine and to locate practitioners, www.functionalmedicine.org.

For information on integrative medicine and to locate practitioners, integrativemedicine.arizona.edu.

Books:

Living a Connected Life: Creating and Maintaining Relationships that Last, Kathleen Brehony, Ph.D.

The Immune Power Personality: 7 Traits You Can Develop to Stay Healthy, Henry Dreher, M.A.

The Dance of Anger, Harriet Lerner, Ph.D.

Super Immunity, Paul Pearsall, Ph.D.

Mind as Healer, Mind as Slayer, Kenneth Pelletier, Ph.D.

Sound Mind, Sound Body, Kenneth Pelletier, Ph.D.

The Survivor Personality, Al Siebert, Ph.D.

Peace, Love & Healing and *Love, Medicine, & Miracles*, Bernie Siegel, M.D., www.berniesiegelmd.com.

The Type C Connection, Lydia Temoshok, Ph.D., and Henry Dreher.

Full Catastrophe Living, Jon Kabat-Zinn, Ph.D.

Books on diet & exercise:

How to Eat, Move and Be Healthy, Paul Chek.

Take Control of Your Health, Joseph Mercola, M.D.

The Schwarzbein Principle: Losing Weight the Healthy Way, Diana Schwarzbein, M.D.

Good Calories/Bad Calories: Fats, Carbs & the Controversial Science of Diet & Health, Gary Taubes.

Chapter Nine

Depression Fact Sheet: See www.upliftprogram.com/depression.

Books:

The Wellness Book: The Comprehensive Guide to Maintaining Health and Treating Stress-Related Illness, Herbert Benson, M.D., and Eileen M Stuart, R.N., M.S.

Minding the Body, Mending the Mind, Joan Borysenko, Ph.D.

Feeling Good, The New Mood Therapy, David Burns, Ph.D.

Ten Days to Self-Esteem, David Burns, Ph.D.

The Feeling Good Handbook: Using the New Mood Therapy in Everyday Life, David Burns, Ph.D.

Mindfulness, Ellen Langer, Ph.D.

Learned Optimism, Martin Seligman, Ph.D.

Chapter Ten

After the Darkest Hour: How Suffering Begins the Journey to Wisdom, Kathleen Brehony, Ph.D.

Man's Search for Meaning, Viktor Frankl M.D., Ph.D.

NOTES

Chapter One

1. M Bambling, "Mind, Body and Heart: Psychotherapy and the Relationship between Mental and Physical Health," *Psychotherapy in Australia*, 12 (2006): 52-59. Also J Astin et al., "Mind-body medicine: state of the science, implications for practice," *Journal of the American Board of Family Practice*, 16 (2003): 131-147.

2. Multiples sources: William Meggs, *The Inflammation Cure* (New York: McGraw-Hill, 2004). F Balkwill et al., "Smoldering and Polarized Inflammation in the Initiation and Promotion of Malignant Disease," *Cancer Cell*, 7 (2005): 211-17. Robert Weinburg, *The Biology of Cancer* (Oxford, UK: Garland Science, 2006). G Stix, "A Malignant Flame," *Scientific American*, July (2007).

Chapter Two

3. R Ader and N Cohen, "Behaviorally Conditioned Immunosuppression," *Psychosomatic Medicine*, 37 (1975): 333-40.

4. D McClelland and C Kirshnit, "The effect of motivational arousal through films on salivary immunoglobulin A," *Psychology & Health*, 2 (1988): 31-52.

5. C Keysers et al., "A touching sight: SII/PV activation during the observation and experience of touch," *Neuron*, 42 (2004): 335-46.

6. Gabor Mate, *When the Body Says No: Understanding the Stress-Disease Connection* (Hoboken, NJ: Wiley, 2003).

7. For a reference on this technique see: M Marinella, "Woltman's Sign of Hypothyroidism," *Hospital Physician*, January (2004): 31-32. Also H Zulewski et al., "Estimation of Tissue Hypothyroidism by a New Clinical Score- Evalua-

tion of Patients with Various Grades of Hypothyroidism and Controls," *Journal of Clinical Endocrinology and Metabolism*, 82 (1997): 771-76.

8. The Remission Project of the Institute of Noetic Sciences (IONS) —this is now available in full online at: www.noetics.org/research/sr/r_biblio.html. Also in print: Brendan O'Regan and Caryle Hirshberg, *Spontaneous Remission: An Annotated Bibliography* (Petaluma, CA: Institute of Noetic Sciences, 1993).

9. Dawson Church, *The Genie in Your Genes: Epigenetic Medicine and the New Biology of Intention* (Santa Rosa, CA: Elite Books, 2007).

10. H Welch and W Burke, "Destined to worry yourself sick," *Atlanta Journal-Constitution*, May 14 (2008): A17.

11. A Gosline, "Me and my genome," *New Scientist*, July 5 (2008): 36-39.

12. Bruce Lipton, *The Biology of Belief: Unleashing the Power of Consciousness, Matter and Miracles* (Santa Rosa, CA: Elite, 2005).

13. Science Daily, "Relaxation Response Can Influence Expression Of Stress-related Genes," *ScienceDaily*, www.sciencedaily.com/releases/2008/07/080701221501.htm.

14. Ernest Rossi, *The Psychobiology of Gene Expression* (New York: W. W. Norton & Company, 2002).

15. G Gerra et al., "Long-term immune-endocrine effects of bereavement: relationships with anxiety levels and mood," *Psychiatry Research*, 121 (2003): 145-58.

16. Science Daily, "Emory Neuroscientists Use Computer Chip To Help Speech-Impaired Patients Communicate," *ScienceDaily*, www.sciencedaily.com/releases/1998/11/981111080706.htm.

17. Bruce Lipton, *The Biology of Belief: Unleashing the Power of Consciousness, Matter and Miracles* (Santa Rosa, CA: Elite, 2005).

18. F Benedetti, "How the Doctor's Words Affect the Patient's Brain," *Evaluation & The Health Professions*, 25 (2002): 369-86.

19. M Brooks, "The power of belief," *New Scientist*, August 23 (2008): 36-39.

20. E Epel et al., "Accelerated Telomere Shortening in Response to Life Stress." *Proceedings of the national Academy of Sciences*, 101 (2004): 17312-315.

21. R von Känel et al., "Effect of Alzheimer Caregiving Stress and Age on Frailty Markers Interleukin-6, C-Reactive Protein, and D-Dimer," *The Journals of Gerontology Series A: Biological Sciences and Medical Sciences*, 61 (2006): 963-69.

22. J Kiecolt-Glaser et al., "Slowing of wound healing by psychological stress," *Lancet*, 346 (1995): 1194-96.

23. E Clays et al., "Associations Between Dimensions of Job Stress and Biomarkers of Inflammation and Infection," *Journal of Occupational and Environmental Medicine*, 47 (2005): 878-83.

24. E Gullette et al., "Effects of Mental Stress on Myocardial Ischemia During Daily Life," *JAMA*, 277 (1997): 1521-6.

25. P Surtees et al., "Psychological distress, major depressive disorder, and risk of stroke," *Neurology*, 70 (2008): 788-94.

26. J Courtney et al., "Stressful life events and the risk of colorectal cancer," *Epidemiology*, 4 (1993): 407-14.

27. ScienceDaily, "Understanding Role of Stress in Just about Everything," *ScienceDaily*, www.sciencedaily.com/releases/2008/01/080108152439.htm.

28. E Reiche et al., "Stress and Depression-Induced Immune Dysfunction: Implications for the Development and Progression of Cancer," *International Review of Psychiatry*, 17 (2005): 515-27. Also E Reiche et al., "Stress, Depression, the Immune System, and Cancer," *Lancet Oncology*, 5 (2004): 617-25. Also Mika Kivimäki of the University of Helsinki has many published studies relating the effects of job stress to cardiovascular disease and other health issues.

29. K Lillberg et al., "Stressful Life Events and Risk of Breast Cancer in 10,808 Women: A Cohort Study," *American Journal of Epidemiology*, 157 (2003): 415-23.

30. S Sephton, R Sapolsky, H Kraemer, and D Spiegel, "Diurnal cortisol rhythm as a predictor of breast cancer survival," *Journal of the National Cancer Institute*, 92 (2001): 994-1000.

31. L Antonova and C Mueller, "Hydrocortisone down-regulates the tumor suppressor gene BRCA1 in mammary cells: a possible molecular link between stress and breast cancer," *Genes, Chromosomes and Cancer*, 47 (2008): 341-52.

32. E yang et al., "Norepinephrine Up-regulates the Expression of Vascular Endothelial Growth Factor, Matrix Metalloproteinase (MMP)-2, and MMP-9 in Nasopharyngeal Carcinoma Tumor Cells," *Cancer Research*, 66 (2006): 10357-64.

33. S Ben-Eliyahu et al., "Stress, NK cells, and cancer: Still a promissory note," *Brain Behavior and Immunity*, 21 (2007): 881-87.

34. K Sastry et al., "Epinephrine Protects Cancer Cells from Apoptosis via Activation of cAMP-dependent Protein Kinase and BAD Phosphorylation," *The Journal of Biological Chemistry*, 282 (2006): 14094-100.

35. A Steptoe et al., "Neuroendocrine and Inflammatory Factors Associated with Positive Affect in Healthy Men and Women: The Whitehall II Study," *American Journal of Epidemiology*, 167 (2008): 96-102.

36. D Vesely et al., "Elimination of up to 80% of human pancreatic adenocarcinomas in athymic mice by cardiac hormones," *In Vivo*, 21 (2007): 445-51.

37. Victor Frankl, *Man's Search for Meaning* (Boston: Beacon, 2006).

38. Lawrence LeShan, *Cancer as a Turning Point* (New York: Plume, 1994).

39. D Spiegel et al., "The Effect of Psychosocial Treatment on Survival of Patients with Metastatic Breast Cancer," *Lancet*, 2 (1989): 888-91.

40. F Fawzy *et al.*, "Malignant Melanoma: Effects of an Early Structured Psychiatric Intervention, Coping, and Affective State on Recurrence and Survival 6 Years Later," *Archives of General Psychiatry*, 50 (1993): 681-89. Also a ten-year follow-up study of the same group. F Fawzy *et al.*, "Malignant Melanoma: Effects of a Brief, Structured Psychiatric Intervention on Survival and Recurrence at 10 Year Follow-up," *Archives of General Psychiatry*, 60 (2003): 100-03.

41. Multiples sources: B Andersen et al., "Psychological, behavioral, and immune changes following a psychological intervention: A clinical trial," *Journal of Clinical Oncology*, 22 (2004): 3570-80. B Andersen et al., "Distress reduction from a psychological intervention contributes to improved health for cancer patients," *Brain, Behavior and Immunity*, 21 (2007): 953-61. B Andersen et al., "Results from an RCT of a psychological intervention for patients with cancer: I. Mechanisms of change," *Journal of Consulting and Clinical Psychology*, 75 (2007): 927-38.

42. L Thornton, B Andersen and W Carson, "Immune, endocrine, and behavioral precursors to breast cancer recurrence: a case-control analysis," *Cancer Immunology, Immunotherapy*, 57 (2008): 1471-81.

43. Science Daily, "Behavioral Program Boosts Antibody That Fights Breast Cancer," *Science Daily*, www.sciencedaily.com/releases/1999/09/990901081334 .htm.

44. J Lackner et al., "Self-Administered Cognitive Behavioral Therapy for Moderate to Severe Irritable Bowel Syndrome: Clinical Efficacy, Tolerability, Feasibility," *Clinical Gastroenterology and Hepatology*, 6 (2008): 899-906.

45. Henry Dreher, *Mind-Body Unity: A New Vision for Mind-Body Science and Medicine* (Baltimore, MD: John's Hopkins University Press, 2003): 194.

46. W Frey et al., "Effect of Stimulus on the chemical composition of human tears," *American Journal of Ophthalmology*, 92 (1981): 559-67.

47. R Dafter, "Why 'Negative' Emotions Can Sometimes Be Positive: The Spectrum Model of Emotions and Their Role in Mind-Body Healing," *Advances: The Journal of Mind-Body Health*, 12 (1996): 6-19.

48. A Grandey et al., "Must "Service with a Smile" Be Stressful? The Moderating Role of Personal Control for American and French Employees," *Journal*

of Applied Psychology, 90 (2005): 893-904. Also A Grandey et al., "Display rules versus display autonomy: Emotion regulation, emotional exhaustion, and task performance in a call center simulation," *Journal of Occupational Health Psychology*, 12 (2007): 301-18.

49. J Burns et al., "Effects of Anger Suppression on Pain Severity and Pain Behaviors Among Chronic Pain Patients: Evaluation of an Ironic Process Model," *Health Psychology*, 24 (2008): 645-52.

50. Lydia Temoshok and Henry Dreher, *The Type C Connection: Mind-Body Link to Cancer and Your Health* (New York: Random House, 1992).

51. S Stern et al., Hopelessness Predicts Mortality in Older Mexican and European Americans," *Psychosomatic Medicine*, 63 (2001): 344-51.

52. Bio-Medicine.org, "Just the expectation of a mirthful laughter experience boosts endorphins 27 percent, HGH 87 percent," Bio-Medicine.org, www. bio-medicine.org/biology-news/Just-the-expectation-of-a-mirthful-laughter -experience-boosts-endorphins-27-percent--HGH-87-percent-2927-1/.

53. S Lewis, "Studying the Biology of Hope: An Interview with Lee S. Berk, DrPH, MPH," *Advances in Mind-Body Medicine*, 22 (2007): 28-31.

Chapter Three

54. Multiple sources: E Reiche et al., "Stress, Depression, the Immune system and Cancer," Lancet, 5 (2004): 617-25. R Schneider et al., "Long-term effects of stress reduction on mortality in persons > or = 55 years of age with systemic hypertension," *The American Journal of Cardiology*, 95 (2005): 1060-4. R Rosmond, "Role of stress in the pathogenesis of metabolic syndrome," *Psychoneuroendocrinology*, 30 (2005): 1-10. C Gorman and A Park, "The Fires Within," *Time*, Feb 23rd (2004).

55. E Clays et al., "Associations between dimensions of job stress and biomarkers of inflammation and infection," *Journal of Occupational and Environmental Medicine*, 47 (2005): 878-83.

56. D Redwood, "Dr. Redwood Interviews Dharma Singh Khalsa, M.D., author of Brain Longevity," www.drredwood.com/interviews/khalsa.shtml. Also Dharma Singh Khalsa, *Brain Longevity* (New York: Warner Books, 1997)

57. N Branan and M Wenner, "Exercising Generates New Brain Cells...And Stress Kills Them Off," *Scientific American Mind*, June/July (2007): 10.

58. R Sapolsky et al., "Hippocampal damage associated with prolonged glucocorticoid exposure in primates," *The Journal of Neuroscience*, 10 (1990): 2897-2902. Also B Stein-Behrens et al., "Stress exacerbates neuron loss and

cytoskeletal pathology in the hippocampus," *The Journal of Neuroscience,* 14 (1994): 5373-5380.

59. Multiple sources: E Reiche et al., "Stress, Depression, the Immune system and Cancer," *Lancet,* 5 (2004): 617-25. E Reiche et al., "Stress and Depression-induced immune dysfunction: implications for the development and progression of cancer," *International Review of Psychiatry,* 17 (2005): 515-27. M Kemeny and M Shedlowski, "Understanding the interaction between psychosocial stress and immune-related diseases: a stepwise progression," *Brain, Behavior and Immunity,* 21 (2007): 1009-18. C Raison and A Miller, "The neuroimmunology of stress and depression," *Seminars in Clinical Neuropsychiatry,* 6 (2001): 277-94. Y Gidron and A Ronson, "Psychosocial factors, biological mediators, and cancer prognosis: a new look at an old story," *Current Opinion in Oncology,* 20 (2008): 386-92.

60. L Dettenborn et al., "Heightened cortisol responses to daily stress in working women at familial risk of breast cancer," *Biological Psychology,* 69 (2005): 167-79.

61. S Sinatra, "Detox that's as easy as breathing," *The Sinatra Health Report,* March (2004).

62. J Shields, "Lymph, lymph glands, and homeostasis," *Lymphology,* 25 (1992): 147-53.

63. Multiple sources: E Holloway and F Ram, "Breathing exercises for asthma," *Cochrane database of systematic reviews,* 1 (2004): CD001277, www.jr2.ox.ac.uk/bandolier/booth/alternat/breathexasthma.html and www.cochrane.org/reviews/en/ab001277.html. M Thomas et al., "Breathing retraining for dysfunctional breathing in asthma: a randomized controlled trial," *Thorax,* 58 (2003): 110-15. M Girodo et al., "Deep diaphragmatic breathing: rehabilitation exercises for the asthmatic patient," *Archives of Physical Medicine and Rehabilitation,* 73 (1992): 717-20.

64. Multiple sources: R Surwit et al., "Stress Management Improves Long-Term Glycemic Control in Type II Diabetes," *Diabetes Care,* 25 (2002): 30-34. S Jablon et al., "Effects of relaxation training on glucose tolerance and diabetic control in type II diabetes," *Applied Psychophysiology and Biofeedback,* 22 (1997): 155-69. R McGinnis et al., "Biofeedback-assisted relaxation in type 2 diabetes," *Diabetes Care,* 28 (2005): 2145-9.

65. S Lazar et al., "Meditation experience is associated with increased cortical thickness," *Neuroreport,* 16 (2005): 1893-97.

66. A Weil, "The Art of Breathing: Proper breathing is the master key to good health," *Dr. Andrew Weil's Self Healing,* May (1998).

67. Two examples include: E Grossman et al., "Breathing-control lowers blood pressure," *Journal of Human Hypertension,* 15 (2001): 263-69. M Shein et al., "Treating hypertension with a device that slows and regularizes breathing: a randomized, double-blind controlled study," *Journal of Human Hypertension,* 15 (2001): 271-78.

68. R Schneider et al., "Long-term effects of stress reduction on mortality in persons > or = 55 years of age with systemic hypertension," *The American Journal of Cardiology,* 95 (2005): 1060-4.

69. L DiCara and N Miller, "Instrumental learning of vasomotor responses by rats: learning to respond differentially in two ears," *Science,* 159 (1968): 1485-6.

70. A Danese et al., "Childhood maltreatment predicts adult inflammation in a life-course study," *Proceedings of the National Academy of Sciences,* 104 (2007): 1319-24.

71. L Schleifer et al., "A hyperventilation theory of job stress and musculoskeletal disorders," *American Journal of Industrial Medicine,* 41 (2002): 420-32.

Chapter Four

72. P Cohen, "Mental gymnastics increase bicep strength," *New Scientist,* Nov (2001): www.newscientist.com/article.ns?id=dn1591.

73. P Fletcher et al., "Brain activity during memory retrieval. The influence of imagery and semantic cueing," *Brain,* 119 (1996): 1587-96. J Ross et al., "The Mind's Eye: Functional MR Imaging Evaluation of Golf Motor Imagery," *American Journal of Neuroradiology,* 24 (2003): 1036-44.

74. Mayo Clinic Health Letter, "Guided Imagery: Enhance Your Healing," *Mayo Clinic Health Letter,* 26 (2008): 6.

75. C Lengacher et al., "Immune Responses to Guided Imagery During Breast Cancer Treatment," *Biological Research for Nursing,* 9 (2008): 205-14.

76. A Pascual-Leone, "The brain that plays music and is changed by it," *Annals of the New York Academy of Sciences,* 930 (2001): 315-29.

77. Piero Ferrucci, *What We May Be: Techniques for Psychological and Spiritual Growth Through Psychosynthesis* (New York: Tarcher/Putnam, 1982).

78. An excellent example of this is found also in this article: M Lacourse et al., "Brain activation during execution and motor imagery of novel and skilled sequential hand movements," *Neuroimage,* 27 (2005): 505-19.

79. Mayo Clinic Health Letter, "Guided Imagery: Enhance Your Healing," *Mayo Clinic Health Letter,* 26 (2008): 6.

80. R Stephens, "Imagery: a strategic intervention to empower clients: Part I—Review of research literature," *Clinical Nurse Specialist*, 7 (1993): 170-4. R Stephens, "Imagery: a strategic intervention to empower clients: Part II—A practical guide," *Clinical Nurse Specialist*, 7 (1993): 235-40. J Lane et al., "Brief meditation training can improve perceived stress and negative mood," *Alternative Therapies in Health and Medicine*, 13 (2007): 38-44.

81. Multiple sources: J Crowther, "Stress management training and relaxation imagery in the treatment of essential hypertension," *Journal of Behavioral Medicine*, 6 (1983): 169-87. V Menzies and S Kim, "Relaxation and guided imagery in Hispanic persons diagnosed with fibromyalgia: a pilot study," *Family & Community Health*, 31 (2008): 204-12. V Menzies et al., "Effects of guided imagery on outcomes of pain, functional status, and self-efficacy in persons diagnosed with fibromyalgia," *Journal of Alternative and Complementary Medicine*, 12 (2006): 23-30. D Carrico et al., "Guided imagery for women with interstitial cystitis: results of a prospective, randomized controlled pilot study," *Journal of Alternative and Complementary Medicine*, 14 (2008): 53-60. L Eller, "Guided imagery interventions for symptom management," *Annual Review of Nursing Research*, 17 (1999): 57-84. J Gruzelier, "A review of the impact of hypnosis, relaxation, guided imagery and individual differences on aspects of immunity and health," *Stress*, 5 (2002): 147-63. D Bazzo and R Moeller, "Imagine this! Infinite uses of guided imagery in women's health," *Journal of Holistic Nursing*, 17 (1999): 317-30. J Weydert et al., "Evaluation of guided imagery as treatment for recurrent abdominal pain in children: a randomized controlled trial," *BMC Pediatrics*, 6 (2006), www.biomedcentral.com/1471-2431/6/29. W Redd et al., "Behavioral intervention for cancer treatment side effects," *Journal of the National Cancer Institute*, 93 (2001): 810-23. L Halpin et al., "Guided imagery in cardiac surgery," *Outcomes Management*, 6 (2002): 132-7. D Tusek et al., "Guided imagery: a significant advance in the care of patients undergoing elective colorectal surgery," *Disease of the Colon and Rectum*, 40 (1997): 172-8. G Antall and D Kresevic, "The use of guided imagery to manage pain in an elderly orthopedic population," *Orthopedic Nursing*, 23 (2004): 335-40. H Yoo et al., "Efficacy of progressive muscle relaxation training and guided imagery in reducing chemotherapy side effects in patients with breast cancer and in improving their quality of life," *Supportive Care in Cancer*, 13 (2005), www.springerlink.com/content/gq7773610t82h3q2/fulltext.html. C Ginandes et al., "Can medical hypnosis accelerate post-surgical wound healing? Results of a clinical trial," *American Journal of Clinical Hypnosis*, 45 (2003): 333-51. S Page et al., "Mental Practice in Chronic Stroke: Results of a randomized, place-bo-controlled trial," *Stroke*, 38 (2007): 1293-97. K Liu et al., "Mental Imagery

for Promoting Relearning for People After Stroke: a Randomized Controlled Study," *Archives of Physical Medicine and Rehabilitation*, 85 (2004): 1403-8. S Richardson, "Effects of Relaxation and Imagery on the Sleep of Critically Ill Adults," *Dimensions of Critical Care Nursing*, 22 (2003): 182-90. H Hall, "Imagery and Cancer," in *Healing Images, the Role of Imagination in Health*, ed. Anees Sheikh (New York, Baywood Publishing Company, Inc., 2003): 408-26.

82. E Trakhtenberg, "The effect of guided imagery on the immune system: a critical review," *International Journal of Neuroscience*, 118 (2008): 839-55.

83. C Wynd, "Guided Health Imagery for Smoking Cessation and Long-Term Abstinence," *Journal of Nursing Scholarship*, 37 (2005): 245-50.

84. M Bambling, "Mind, Body, and Heart: Psychotherapy and the Relationship between Mental and Physical Health," *Psychotherapy in Australia*, 12 (2006): 52-59.

85. S Sivasankara et al., "The effect of a six week program of yoga and meditation on brachial artery reactivity: do psychosocial interventions affect vascular tone?" *Clinical Cardiology*, 29 (2006): 393-8.

86. R Schneider et al., "Long-term effects of stress reduction on mortality in persons > or = 55 years of age with systemic hypertension," *American Journal of Cardiology*, 95 (2005): 1060-64.

87. Martin Rossman, *Guided Imagery for Self-Healing* (Tiburon, CA: New World Library, 2000).

88. D Schwabb et al., "A Study of Efficacy and Cost-effectiveness of Guided Imagery as a Portable, Self-administered, Presurgical Intervention Delivered by a Health Plan," *Advances in Mind-Body Medicine*, 22 (2007): 8-14.

89. D Schwabb et al., "A Study of Efficacy and Cost-effectiveness of Guided Imagery as a Portable, Self-administered, Presurgical Intervention Delivered by a Health Plan," *Advances in Mind-Body Medicine*, 22 (2007): 8-14.

90. C Baird and L Sands, "A Pilot Study of the Effectiveness of Guided Imagery with Progressive Muscle Relaxation to Reduce Chronic Pain and Mobility Difficulties of Osteoarthritis," *Pain Management Nursing: The Official Journal of the American Society of Pain Management Nurses*, 5 (2004): 97-104.

91. E Watanabe et al., "Effects among healthy subjects of the duration of regularly practicing a guided imagery program," *BMC Complementary and Alternative Medicine*, 20 (2005), www.biomedcentral.com/1472-6882/5/21.

92. O Carl Simonton and Stephanie Matthews-Simonton, *Getting Well Again: A Step-By-Step Self help Guide to Overcoming Cancer for Patients and Their Families* (Los Angeles: Jeremy P. Tarcher, 1978).

93. Jeanne Achterberg and G Frank Lawlis, *Bridges of the bodymind: Behavioral approaches to health care* (Champaign, Illinois: Institute for Personal-

ity and Ability Testing, Inc. 1980), J Achterberg et al., "Use of Imagery in the Treatment of Cardiovascular Disorders," in *Healing Images, the Role of Imagination in Health,* ed. Anees Sheikh (New York, Baywood Publishing Company, Inc., 2003): 300-11. J Achterberg et al., "Effect of immune system imagery of secretory IgA," *Biofeedback and Self-Regulation,* 15 (1990): 317-33,

94. Deirdre Brigham, *Imagery for Getting Well* (New York: Norton, 1994).

95. O Carl Simonton and Stephanie Matthews-Simonton, *Getting Well Again: A Step-By-Step Self help Guide to Overcoming Cancer for Patients and Their Families* (Los Angeles: Jeremy P. Tarcher, 1978).

96. *Getting Well* program. This program no longer exists but the Resource Guide lists some current programs that are available.

97. Multiple sources: J Taal and J Krop, "Imagery in the Treatment of Trauma," in *Healing Images, the Role of Imagination in Health,* ed. Anees Sheikh (New York, Baywood Publishing Company, Inc., 2003): 396-407. J Davis, "Exposure, Relaxation, and Rescripting Treatment for Trauma-Related Nightmares," *Journal of Trauma and Dissociation,* 7 (2006): 5-18. B Krakow et al., "Imagery rehearsal therapy for chronic nightmares in sexual assault survivors with posttraumatic stress disorder: a randomized controlled trial," *JAMA,* 286 (2001): 537-45. R Lysaght and E Bodenhamer, "The use of relaxation training to enhance functional outcomes in adults with traumatic head injuries," *American Journal of Occupational Therapy,* 44 (1990): 797-802. J Wies et al., "Imagery: Its History and Use in the Treatment of Posttraumatic Stress Disorder," in *Healing Images, the Role of Imagination in Health,* ed. Anees Sheikh (New York, Baywood Publishing Company, Inc., 2003): 381-95.

98. John McCrone, *Going Inside: A Tour Round a Single Moment of Consciousness* (London: Faber & Faber, 1999) and Jeffrey Gray, *Consciousness: Creeping up on the Hard Problem* (Oxford: Oxford University Press, 2004).

99. J Raymond et al., "The effects of alpha/theta neurofeedback on personality and mood," *Brain Research. Cognitive Brain Research,* 23 (2005): 287-92. E Baehr et al., "The Clinical Use of An Alpha Asymmetry Protocol in the Neurofeedback Training of Depression: Two Case Studies," *Journal of Neurotherapy,* 4 (2001): 11-18. E Saxby and E Peniston, "Alpha-theta brainwave neurofeedback training: an effective treatment for male and female alcoholics with depressive symptoms," *Journal of Clinical Psychology,* 51 (1995): 685-93. T Sokhadze et al., "EEG Biofeedback as a Treatment for Substance Use Disorders: Review, Rating of Efficacy, and Recommendations for Further Research," *Applied Psychophysiology and Biofeedback,* 33 (2008): 1-28. S Kayiran et al., "Neurofeedback in Fibromyalgia Syndrome," *Agri,* 19 (2007): 47-53. K Dohrmann et al., "Neurofeedback for treating tinnitus," *Progress in Brain Research,* 166 (2007):

473-85. P Friel, "EEG biofeedback in the treatment of attention deficit hyperactivity disorder," *Alternative Medicine Review*, 12 (2007): 146-51. M Sterman and T Egner, "Foundation and practice of neurofeedback for the treatment of epilepsy," *Applied Psychophysiology and Biofeedback*, 31 (2006): 21-35. H Heinrich et al., "Annotation: neurofeedback – train your brain to train behavior," *Journal of Child Psychology and Psychiatry*, 48 (2007): 3-16. J Becerra et al., "Follow-up study of learning-disabled children treated with neurofeedback or placebo," *Clinical EEG and Neuroscience*, 37 (2006): 198-203. G Rozelle and T Budzynski, "Neurotherapy for stroke rehabilitation: a single case study," *Biofeedback and Self-Regulation*, 20 (1995): 211-28. D Hammond, "Neurofeedback with anxiety and affective disorders," *Child and Adolescent Psychiatric Clinics of North America*, 14 (2005): 105-23, vii.

Chapter Five

100. C Kenneally, "The Food Of Love – In Six Courses," *New Scientist*, August 28 (2008): 47.

101. Wikipedia, "History of Music," en.wikipedia.org/wiki/History_of_music.

102. Wikipedia, "Water organ," en.wikipedia.org/wiki/Hydraulis.

103. Multiple sources: L Bernardi et al., "Cardiovascular, cerebrovascular and respiratory changes induced by different types of music in musicians and non-musicians: the importance of silence," *Heart*, 92 (2006): 445-52. S Evers et al., "The cerebral haemodynamics of music perception. A transcranial Doppler study," *Brain*, 122 (1999): 75-85. E Altenmuller, "Brain electrical correlates of cerebral music processing in the human," *European Archives of Psychiatry and Neurological Sciences*, 235 (1986): 342-54. S Iakovides et al., "Psychophysiology and psychoacoustics of music: Perception of complex sound in normal subjects and psychiatric patients," *BioMed Central: Annals of General Psychiatry*, 3 (2004): www.annals-general-psychiatry.com/content/3/1/6. S Koelsch et al., "Effects of unexpected chords and of performer's expression on brain responses and electrodermal activity, *PLoS One*, 3 (2008): e2631, www.plosone.org/article/info:doi%2F10.1371%2Fjournal.pone.0002631. S Leardi et al, "Randomized clinical trial examining the effect of music therapy in stress response to day surgery," *The British Journal of Surgery*, 94 (2007): 943-7.

104. Mitchell Gaynor, *The Healing Power of Sound: Recovery from Life-Threatening Illness Using Sound, Voice and Music* (Boston: Shambala Publications, 1999).

105. D Tzvetkov and R Tzanev, "Vibrational effects on fatty acid composition of organ and cell membrane lipids," *La medicina del lavoro*, 82 (1991): 3-10.

106. K Tsen et al., "Selective inactivation of human immunodeficiency virus with subpicosecond near-infrared laser pulses," *IOP: Journal of Physics: Condensed Matter*, 25 (2008): 252205, www.iop.org/EJ/article/0953 -8984/20/25/252205/cm8_25_252205.html.

107. R McCraty et al., "Music Enhances the Effect of Positive Emotional States on Salivary IgA," *Stress Medicine*, 12 (1996): 167-75.

108. Multiple sources: E Labbe et al., "Coping with stress: the effectiveness of different types of music," *Applied Psychophysiology and Biofeedback*, 32 (2007): 163-8. S Wang et al., "Music and preoperative anxiety: a randomized, controlled study," *Anesthesia and Analgesia*, 94 (2002): 1489-94. E Yilmaz et al, "Music decreases anxiety and provides sedation in extracorporeal shock wave lithotripsy," *Urology*, 61 (2003): 282-6. Also see endnote #3 for other references. The American Music Therapy Association website can be found at www. musictherapy.org/. M Rider et al., "The effect of music, therapy, and relaxation on adrenal corticosteroids and the re-entrainment of circadian rhythms," *Journal of Music Therapy*, 22 (1985): 46-58. J Smith and C Joyce, "Mozart versus new age music: relaxation states, stress, and the ABC relaxation theory," *Journal of Music Therapy*, 41 (2004): 215-24. C Boyd-Brewer and R McAffrey, "Vibroacoustic sound therapy improves pain management and more," *Holistic Nursing Practice*, 18 (2004): 111-8.

109. Judith Orloff, *Positive Energy: 10 Extraordinary Prescriptions for Transforming Fatigue, Stress, and Fear into Vibrance, Strength, and Love* (New York: Random House, 2004). Also M Balick and R Lee, "The Power Of Sound: Ethnomedical Tradition And Modern Science," *Alternative Therapies in Health and Medicine*, 9 (2003): 96-99.

110. Multiple sources: A Ferrer, "The effect of live music on decreasing anxiety in patients undergoing chemotherapy treatment," *Journal of Music Therapy*, 44 (2007): 242-55. U Nilsson et al., "Stress reduction and analgesia in patients exposed to calming music postoperatively: a randomized controlled trial," *European Journal of Anaesthesiology*, 22 (2005): 96-102. R McCaffrey and E Freeman, "Effect of music on chronic osteoarthritis pain in older people," *Journal of Advanced Nursing*, 44 (2003): 517-24. S Siedliecki and M Good, "Effect of music on power, pain, depression and disability," *Journal of Advanced Nursing*, 54 (2006): 553-62. G Stefano et al., "Music alters constitutively expressed opiate and cytokine processes in listeners," *Medical Science Monitor*, 10 (2004): MS18-27, journals.indexcopernicus.com/fulltxt.php?ICID=11690. M Boso et al, "Neurophysiology and neurobiology of the musical experience," *Functional Neurology*, 21 (2006): 187-91. L Harmat et al., "Music improves sleep quality in students," *Journal of Advanced Nursing*, 62 (2008): 327-35.

S Hanser and S Mandel, "The effects of music therapy in cardiac healthcare," *Cardiology in Review*, 13 (2005): 18-23. J White, "Effects of relaxing music on cardiac autonomic balance and anxiety after acute myocardial infarction," *American Journal of Critical Care*, 8 (1999): 220-30.

111. T Särkämö et al., "Music listening enhances cognitive recovery and mood after middle cerebral artery stroke," *Brain*, 131 (2008): 866-76.

112. C Emery et al., "Short-term effects of exercise and music on cognitive performance among participants in a cardiac rehabilitation program," *Heart & Lung: the Journal of Acute and Critical Care*, 32 (2003): 368-73.

113. Don Campbell, *The Mozart Effect: Tapping the Power of Music to Heal the Body, Strengthen the Mind, and Unlock the Creative Spirit* (New York: HarperCollins, 2001).

114. Y Qin et al., "Biochemical and physiological changes in plants as a result of different sonic exposures," *Ultrasonics*, 41 (2003): 407-11.

115. M Penner, "Classic Year Promised as Mozart is heard on the grapevine," *Times Online*, 2005, www.timesonline.co.uk/tol/news/world/europe/article570831.ece. Also N Martinelli, "Grape Expectations: Vines May Love Vivaldi," *Wired*, 2007, www.wired.com/science/discoveries/news/2007/06/music_and_wine.

116. J Pantaleone, "Synchronization of metronomes," *American Journal of Physics*, 70 (2002): 992-1000.

117. Multiple sources: K Kojima et al., "Role of the community effect of cardiomyocyte in the entrainment and reestablishment of stable beating rhythms," *Biochemical and Biophysical Research Communications*, 351 (2006): 209-15. S Strogatz and I Stewart, "Coupled oscillators and biological synchronization," *Scientific American*, 269 (1993): 102-9. J Anumonwo et al., "Phase resetting and entrainment of pacemaker activity in single sinus nodal cells," *Circulation Research*, 68 (1991): 1138-53.

118. J White, "Effects of relaxing music on cardiac autonomic balance and anxiety after acute myocardial infarction," *American Journal of Critical Care*, 8 (1999): 220-30.

119. X Liu et al., "Comparison of stress response between mental tasks and white noise exposure," *Journal of Physiological Anthropology*, 26 (2007): 165-71. X Teng et al., "The effect of Music on Hypertensive Patients," *Conference proceedings: Engineering in Medicine and Biology Society*, 2007: 4649-51. E Grossman et al.," Breathing-control lowers blood pressure," *Journal of Human Hypertension*, 15 (2001): 263-69. [The Grossman study used breathing with interactive music]

120. K Allen et al., "Normalization of hypertensive responses during ambulatory surgical stress by perioperative music," *Psychosomatic Medicine*, 63 (2001): 487-92. Also S Barnason et al., "The effects of music interventions on anxiety in the patient after coronary artery bypass grafting," *Heart & Lung: the Journal of Acute and Critical Care*, 24 (1995): 124-32.

121. E Tasali et al., "Slow-Wave sleep and the risk of type II diabetes in humans," *PNAS*, 105 (2008): 1044-49.

122. Memorial Sloan-Kettering: www.mskcc.org/mskcc/html/69308.cfm. The University of Texas MD Anderson Cancer Center: Music Therapy: www.mdanderson.org/departments/wellness/dIndex.cfm?pn=7E34C910-EDEF-44FC-A5DBE5C455CE67C0.

123. D Aldridge, "The Music of the Body: Music Therapy in Medical Settings," *Advances, The Journal of Mind-Body Health*, 9 (1993): 17-35.

124. Ibid.

125. M Balick and R Lee, "The Power Of Sound: Ethnomedical Tradition And Modern Science," *Alternative Therapies in Health and Medicine*, 9 (2003): 96-99.

126. M Koch, Z Kain et al., "The sedative and analgesic sparing effect of music," *Anesthesiology*, 89 (1998): 300-6. Also D Lee et al., "Relaxation music decreases the dose of patient-controlled sedation during colonoscopy: a prospective randomized controlled trial," *Gastrointestinal Endoscopy*, 55 (2002): 33-6.

127. E Ikonomidou et al., "Effect of Music on Vital Signs and Postoperative Pain," *Association of periOperative Registered Nurses*, 80 (2004): 269-78.

128. W Poole, *The Heart of Healing* (Atlanta: Turner Publishing, Inc., 1993).

129. C Pacchetti et al., "Active Music Therapy in Parkinson's Disease: An Integrative Method for Motor and Emotional Rehabilitation," *Psychosomatic Medicine*, 62 (2000): 386-93.

130. Robert Tusler, *Music: Catalyst for Healing* (Alkmaar, Netherlands: Drukkerij Krijgsman, 1991).

131. Masaru Emoto, *The Hidden Messages in Water* (Hillsboro, Oregon: Beyond Words Publishing, 2004).

132. Judith Orloff, *Positive Energy: 10 Extraordinary Prescriptions for Transforming Fatigue, Stress, and Fear into Vibrance, Strength, and Love* (New York: Random House, 2004).

133. H Berg, "Possibilities and problems of low frequency weak electromagnetic fields in cell biology," *Bioelectrochemistry and Bioenergetics*, 38 (1995):

153-59. C Bassett, "Low energy pulsing electromagnetic fields modify biological processes," *Bioessays*, 6 (2005): 36-42. Frank Barnes and Ben Greenebaum, ed., *Handbook of biological effects of electromagnetic fields, 3rd Edition* (Boca Raton, Fl: CRC Press, 2006).

134. W Knight, "Cellphones 'should not be given to children'," *New Scientist*, Jan (2005): www.newscientist.com/article.ns?id=dn6872. R Herberman, "The Case for Precaution in the Use of Cell Phones Advice from University of Pittsburgh Cancer Institute Based on Advice from an International Expert Panel," *University of Pittsburgh Cancer Institute*, www.upci.upmc.edu/news/upci_news/2008/072308_celladvisory.html. Commenting of the REFLEX report is the NIRMED statement, "Genotoxic and Cytotoxic Research Results and their Relevance for the Estimation of possible Adverse Health Effects caused by Low Level Electromagnetic Fields," *NIRMED*, www.nirmed.de/downloads/finalnirmedreflex.pdf.

135. R Le Scouarnec et al., "Use of binaural beat tapes for treatment of anxiety: a pilot study of tape preference and outcomes," *Alternative therapies in health and medicine*, 7 (2001): 58-63.

136. J Lane et al., "Binaural auditory beats affect vigilance performance and mood," *Physiology and Behavior*, 63 (1998): 249-52.

137. R Padmanabhan et al., "A prospective, randomised, controlled study examining binaural beat audio and pre-operative anxiety in patients undergoing general anaesthesia for day case surgery," *Anaesthesia*, 60 (2005): 874-7.

138. D Schwartz and P Taylor, "Human auditory steady state responses to binaural and monaural beats," *Clinical Neurophysiology*, 116 (2005): 658-68.

139. H Wahbeh et al., "Binaural beat technology in humans: a pilot study to assess psychologic and physiologic effects," *Journal of Alternative and Complementary Medicine*, 13 (2007): 25-32. H Wahbeh et al., "Binaural beat technology in humans: a pilot study to assess neuropsychologic, physiologic, and electroencephalographic effects," *Journal of Alternative and Complementary Medicine*, 13 (2007): 199-206.

140. The Monroe Institute: www.monroeinstitute.com/.

141. Alfred Tomatis, *Why Mozart?* (Editions Fixot, 1991). Also Pierre Sollier, *Listening for Wellness: An Introduction to the Tomatis Method* (Walnut Creek, CA: The Mozart Center Press, 2005).

142. Mitchell Gaynor, *The Healing Power of Sound: Recovery from Life-Threatening Illness Using Sound, Voice and Music* (Boston: Shambala Publications, 1999): 143-6.

143. G Avanzini, ed., "The Neurosciences and Music II: From Perception to Performance," *Annals of the New York Academy of Sciences,* 1060 (2006).

144. Mitchell Gaynor, *The Healing Power of Sound: Recovery from Life-Threatening Illness Using Sound, Voice and Music* (Boston: Shambala Publications, 1999): 136.

145. Ibid: 146-7.

146. Multiple sources: S Ohno and M Ohno, "The all pervasive principle of repetitious recurrence governs not only coding sequence construction but also human endeavor in musical composition," *Immunogenetics,* 24 (1986): 71-8. S Ohno, "Repetition as the essence of life on this earth: music and genes," *Haematology and Blood Transfusion,* 31 (1987): 511-8. Also A Sanchez-Sousa et al., "The making of "The Genoma Music"," *Revista Iberoamericana de Micologia,* 22 (2005): 242-8.

147. Multiple sources: B Bittman et al., "Composite effects of group drumming music therapy on modulation of neuroendocrine-immune parameters in normal subjects," *Alternative Therapies in Health and Medicine,* 7 (2001): 38-47. M Wachi, B Bittman et al., "Recreational music-making modulates natural killer cell activity, cytokines, and mood states in corporate employees," *Medical Science Monitor,* 13 (2007): CR57-70, www.medscimonit.com/fulltxt .php?ICID=473761. B Bittman et al., "Recreational music-making: an integrative group intervention for reducing burnout and improving mood states in first year associate degree nursing students: insights and economic impact," *International Journal of Nursing Education Scholarship,* 1 (2004): Article 12, www.bepress.com/ijnes/vol1/iss1/art12.

148. Dharma Singh Khalsa, *Brain Longevity: The Breakthrough Medical Program That Improves Your Mind and Memory.* (Time Warner, 1999).

149. A Kumar et al., "Music therapy increases serum melatonin levels in patients with Alzheimer's disease," *Alternative Therapies in Health and Medicine,* 5 (1999): 49-57.

150. Plato, Allan Bloom, trans., *The Republic of Plato* (New York: Basic Books, 1991).

151. P Cook, 'Music, Imagery, and Healing," in *Healing Images, the Role of Imagination in Health,* ed. Anees Sheikh (New York, Baywood Publishing Company, Inc., 2003): 115-38.

152. Don Campbell, *The Mozart Effect: Tapping the Power of Music to Heal the Body, Strengthen the Mind, and Unlock the Creative Spirit* (New York: HarperCollins, 2001).

Chapter Six

153 Emmett Miller, *Deep Healing: The Essence of Mind/Body Medicine* (Carlsbad, Ca: Hay House, 1997).

154. Betty Edwards, *Drawing on the Right Side of the Brain* (Los Angeles: Tarcher, 1989).

155. Deirdre Brigham, *Imagery for Getting Well* (New York: Norton, 1994).

156. Lawrence LeShan, *Beyond Technique: Psychotherapy for the 21ˢᵗ Century* (Northvale, NJ: Jason Aronson, Inc., 1996).

157. J Mirowsky and C Ross, "Creative Work and Health," *Journal of Health and Social Behavior*, 48 (2007): 385-403.

158. L Neergaard, "Nap without guilt: It boosts sophisticated memory," *The Guardian*, Nov. 24 (2008): www.guardian.co.uk/uslatest/story/0,,-8075391,00 .html.

159. N Hamilton et al., "Fibromyalgia: The Role of Sleep in Affect and in Negative Event Reactivity and Recovery," *Health Psychology*, 27 (2008): 490-94.

160. J Davidson et al., "Growth hormone and cortisol secretion in relation to sleep and wakefulness," *Journal of Psychiatry and Neuroscience*, 16 (1991): 96-102.

161. S Yoo et al., "The human emotional brain without sleep—a prefrontal amygdala disconnect," *Current Biology*, 17 (2007): R877-R878.

162. Ernest Rossi, *The Psychobiology of Mind-Body Healing* (New York: W. W. Norton & Company, 1993): 205.

163. The Keirsey Temperament Scale. www.keirsey.com/.

164. Mihaly Csikszentmihalyi, *Finding Flow: The Psychology of Engagement with Everyday Life* (New York: Basic Books, 1997).

165. Mihaly Csikszentmihalyi, *Finding Flow: The Psychology of Engagement with Everyday Life* (New York: Basic Books, 1997), 8.

166. US Geological Survey, "Historical Earthquakes," San Fernando, California, earthquake.usgs.gov/regional/states/events/1971_02_09.php. Wikipedia, "1971 San Fernando Earthquake," en.wikipedia.org/wiki/1971_San_Fernando_earthquake.

Chapter Seven

167. Wikipedia, "MS Explorer," en.wikipedia.org/wiki/MS_Explorer.

168. Conversations with Doctors Felitti and Anda.

169. V Felitti, R Anda et al., "Relationship of childhood abuse and household dysfunction to many of the leading causes of death in adults. The Adverse Childhood Experiences (ACE) Study," *American Journal of Preventive Medicine,* 14 (1998): 245-58.

170. J Kaufman et al., "Social supports and serotonin transporter gene moderate depression in maltreated children," *Proceedings of the National Academy of Sciences,* 101 (2004): 17316-21.

171. R Cohen et al., "Violence, Abuse and Asthma in Puerto Rican Children," *American Journal of Respiratory and Critical Care Medicine,* 178 (2008): 453-59.

172. J Pennebaker and C Chung, "Expressive writing, emotional upheavals, and health," in *Foundations of Health Psychology,* ed. Howard Friedman and Roxane Silver (New York: Oxford University Press, 2007), 263-84.

173. Henry Dreher, *Mind-Body Unity: A New Vision for Mind-Body Science and Medicine* (Baltimore, MD: John's Hopkins University Press, 2003).

174. *Ibid*: 214-15.

175. J Kelley et al., "Health effects of emotional disclosure in rheumatoid arthritis patients," *Health Psychology,* 16 (1997): 331-40.

176. This chapter title is based upon a book by Deena Metzger, *Writing for Your Life* (New York: HarperCollins, 2007).

177. Stephen Lepore and Joshua Smyth, ed., *The Writing Cure: How Expressive Writing Promotes Health and Emotional Well-Being* (Washington, D.C.: American Psychological Association, 2002).

178. J Smyth et al., "Effects of writing about stressful experiences on symptom reduction in patients with asthma or rheumatoid arthritis: a randomized trial," *JAMA,* 281 (1999): 1304-9.

179. Pennebaker has conducted at least a dozen studies on these topics published in multiple journals.

180. P Graves et al., "Temperament as a potential predictor of mortality: Evidence from a 41-year prospective study," *Journal of Behavioral Medicine,* 17 (1994): 111-26.

181. K Klein and A Boals, "Expressive writing can increase working memory capacity," *Journal of experimental psychology. General,* 130 (2001): 520-33. Also M Yogo and S Fujihara, "Working memory capacity can be improved by expressive writing: a randomized experiment in a Japanese sample," *British Journal of Health Psychology,* 13 (2008): 77-80.

182. T Simonite, "Stabbed in Translation," *New Scientist,* December 17th, 2007, www.newscientist.com/blog/technology/labels/internet.html.

183. M Lumley et al., "The effects of written emotional disclosure among repressive and alexithymic people," in *The Writing Cure: How Expressive Writing Promotes Health and Emotional Well-Being*, ed. Stephen Lepore and Joshua Smyth (Washington, D.C.: American Psychological Association, 2002): 75.

184. I first became familiar with this reference in Goldstein and Goldstein, *"How We Know: An Exploration of the Scientific Process* (New York: Da Capo Press, 1978), 192. The quote about Helen's life is from Helen Keller, *The Story of My Life* (New York: Bantam Classics, 1990).

185. I Wickramasekera, "Secrets kept from the mind but not the body or behavior," *Advances in Mind/Body Medicine*, 14 (1998): 81-132. This is just one of many references from an abundance of evidence in psychophysiology research.

186. A Lange et al., "Interapy: A Model for Therapeutic Writing Through the Internet," in *The Writing Cure: How Expressive Writing Promotes Health and Emotional Well-Being*, ed. Stephen Lepore and Joshua Smyth (Washington, D.C.: American Psychological Association, 2002), 215-38.

187. R Norris and S Bauer-Wu, "Being mindful, easing suffering." *Journal of Palliative Medicine*, 10 (2007): 261-2.

188. Barbara Herrick, *The Blackberry Tea Club: Women in Their Glory Years* (Boston: Conari Press, 2004).

189. Gabriele Lusser Rico, *Writing the Natural Way* (New York: JP Tarcher, 2000).

190. S Lutgendorf and P Ullrich, "Cognitive Processing, Disclosure, And Health: Psychological And Physiological Mechanisms," in *The Writing Cure: How Expressive Writing Promotes Health and Emotional Well-Being*, ed. Stephen Lepore and Joshua Smyth (Washington, D.C.: American Psychological Association, 2002), 177-96. Also P Tomich and V Helgeson, "Is Finding Something Good in the Bad Always Good? Benefit Finding Among Women With Breast Cancer," *Health Psychology* 23 (2004): 16-23.

191. Multiple sources: A Stanton et al., "The first year after breast cancer diagnosis: hope and coping strategies as predictors of adjustment," *Psychooncology*, 11 (2002): 93-102. A Stanton et al., "Coping with a breast cancer diagnosis: a prospective study," *Health Psychology*, 12 (1993): 16-23. A Stanton et al., "Emotionally expressive coping predicts psychological and physical adjustment to breast cancer," *Journal of Consulting and Clinical Psychology*, 68 (2000): 875-82. A Stanton et al., "Randomized, controlled trial of written emotional expression and benefit finding in breast cancer patients," *Journal of Clinical Oncology*, 20 (2002): 4160-68.

192. C Carver and M Antoni, "Finding benefit in breast cancer the year after diagnosis predicts better adjustment 5 to 8 years after diagnosis," *Health Psychology*, 23 (2004): 595-8.

193. L King, "Gain Without Pain? Expressive Writing and Self-Regulation," in *The Writing Cure: How Expressive Writing Promotes Health and Emotional Well-Being*, ed. Stephen Lepore and Joshua Smyth (Washington, D.C.: American Psychological Association, 2002), 119-34.

194. R Emmons and M McCullough, "Counting blessings versus burdens: Experimental studies of gratitude and subjective well-being," *Journal of Personality and Social Psychology*, 84 (2003): 377-89. J Froh et al., "Gratitude and subjective well-being in early adolescence: Examining gender differences," *Journal of Adolescence*, August (2008): Epub ahead of print at: doi:10.1016/j/adolescence.2008.06.006. T Kashdan et al., "Gratitude and hedonic and eudaimonic well-being in Vietnam war veterans," *Behavior Research and Therapy*, 44 (2006): 177-99.

195. X Liu et al., "Rapid Eye Movement Sleep in Relation to Overweight in Children and Adolescents," *Archives of General Psychiatry*, 65 (2008): 924-32.

196. Stuart Hameroff, M.D., Professor, Departments of Anesthesiology and Psychology, University of Arizona at Tucson, NICABM presentation (2005): 257.

197. Rosalind Cartwright and Lynne Lamberg, *Crisis Dreaming: Using Your Dreams to Solve Your Problems* (Lincoln, NE: ASJA Press, 2000).

198. B Dossey, "On Holistic Nursing, Healing Rituals, and Florence Nightingale," *Network*, 17 (2001): 8-14.

Chapter Eight

199. Paul Pearsall, *Superimmunity* (New York: McGraw-Hill, 1987): 381-83.

200. M Watson et al., "Influence of psychological response on breast cancer survival: 10-year follow-up of a population-based cohort," *European Journal of Cancer*, 41 (2005): 1665-6.

201. M Visintainer et al., "Tumor rejection in rats after inescapable or escapable shock," *Science*, 216 (1982): 437-39.

202. E Langer and J Rodin, "The effects of choice and enhanced responsibility for the aged: A field experiment in an institutional setting," *Journal of Personality and Social Psychology*, 34 (1976): 191-198.

203. S Kobasa et al., "Personality and Constitution as Mediators in the Stress-Illness Relationship," *Journal of Health and Social Behavior,* 22 (1981): 368-78.

204. M Watson et al., "Influence of psychological response on breast cancer survival: 10-year follow-up of a population-based cohort," *European Journal of Cancer,* 41 (2005): 1665-6.

205. M Pessiglione et al., "Subliminal Instrumental Conditioning Demonstrated in the Human Brain," *Neuron,* 59 (2008): 561-67.

206. B Levy, J Hausdorf et al., "Reducing Cardiovascular Stress with Positive Self-Stereotypes of Aging," *The Journals of Gerontology Series B: Psychological Sciences and Social Sciences,* 55 (2000): 205-13.

207. Better Health, "Plants Make Office Happy," *Atlanta Journal-Constitution,* June 11 (2008): K2.

208. Albert Marchetti, *Beating the Odds: Alternative Treatments That Have Worked Miracles Against Cancer* (New York: St. Martin's Press, 1994).

209. Ernest Rossi, *The Psychobiology of Gene Expression* (New York: W. W. Norton & Company, 2002).

210. Jason Theodosakis, *Maximizing the Arthritis Cure: A Step-by-Step Program to Faster, Stronger Healing During Any Stage of the Cure* (New York: St. Martin's Press, 1998).

211. R Levenson et al. "Voluntary facial action generates emotion-specific autonomic nervous system activity," *Psychophysiology,* 4 (1990): 363-384.

212. Al Siebert, *The Survivor Personality* (Portland, OR: Practical Psychology Press, 1994), 4.

213. R Levenson et al. "Voluntary facial action generates emotion-specific autonomic nervous system activity," *Psychophysiology,* 4 (1990): 363-384.

214. L Berk et al., "Modulation of neuroimmune parameters during the eustress of humor-associated mirthful laughter," *Alternative Therapies in Health and Medicine,* 7 (2001): 62-72, 74-6. Also L Berk et al., "Mirthful Laughter, as Adjunct Therapy in Diabetic Care, Attenuates Catecholamines, Inflammatory Cytokines, C - reactive protein, and Myocardial Infarction Occurrence," European Preventive Cardiology Meeting, May (2007).

215. Multiple sources: M Bennett et al., "The effect of mirthful laughter on stress and natural killer cell activity," *Alternative Therapies in Health and Medicine,* 9 (2003): 38-45. R Parse, "Laughing and Health: a study using Parse's research method," *Nursing Science Quarterly,* 7 (1994): 55-64. L Berk et al., Neuroendocrine and stress hormone changes during mirthful laughter," *The American Journal of the Medical Sciences,* 298 (1989): 390-6.

216. A Sahakian and W Frishman, "Humor and the Cardiovascular System," *Alternative Therapies in Health and Medicine*, 13 (2007): 56-58.

217. M Miller et al., "Impact of cinematic viewing on endothelial function," *Heart*, 92 (2006): 261-62.

218. S Tan et al., "Mirthful laughter an effective adjunct in cardiac rehabilitation," *Canadian Journal of Cardiology*, 13 (1997): supplement, 190. M Balick and R Lee, "The Role of Laughter in Traditional Medicine and it's Relevance to the Clinical Setting: Healing with Ha!" *Alternative Therapies in Health and Medicine*, 9 (2003): 88-91.

219. M Miller et al., "Impact of cinematic viewing on endothelial function," *Heart*, 92 (2006): 261-62.

220. P Wooten, "An Interview with William Fry Jr., M.D.," *Journal of Nursing Jocularity*, 4 (1994): 46-47.

221. W Fry, "Mirth and the human cardiovascular system," in *The Study of Humor*, ed. Harvey Mindess and Joy Turek (Los Angeles: Antioch University Press, 1979).

222. T Atsumi et al., "Pleasant feeling from watching comical video enhances free radical-scavenging capacity in human whole saliva," *Journal of Psychosomatic Research*, 56 (2004): 377-9.

223. S Yoshino and E Mukai, "Neuroendocrine-immune system in patients with rheumatoid arthritis," *Journal of Modern Rheumatology*, 13 (2003): 193-98. E Choy, "Interleukin 6 receptor as a target for the treatment of rheumatoid arthritis," *Annals of Rheumatic Disease*, 62 (2003): ii68-ii69.

224. Watchtower Bible and Tract Society, "Facing Illness with a Sense of Humor," *Awake*, April 22 (2005): 26-27.

225. Madan Kataria, *Laugh for No Reason* (Madhuri International, 2002).

226. M Reeves and A Rafferty, "Healthy Lifestyle Characteristics Among Adults in the United States, 2000," *Archives of Internal Medicine*, 165 (2005): 854-57.

227. G Amersbach, "Beyond the Myths of Aging," *Harvard Public Health Review*, Fall 2000, www.hsph.harvard.edu/review/review_2000/featureaging.html.

228. J Blumenthal et al., "Exercise and Pharmacotherapy in the Treatment of Major Depressive Disorder," *Psychosomatic Medicine*, 69 (2007): 587-96.

229. A Naska et al., "Siesta in Healthy Adults and Coronary Mortality in the General Population," *Archives of Internal Medicine*, 167 (2007): 296-301.

230. Lydia Temoshok and Henry Dreher, *The Type C Connection* (New York: Random House, 1992) 390.

231. Stephen Post and Jill Neimark, *Why Good Things Happen to Good People: How to Live a Longer, Healthier, Happier Life by the Simple Act of Giving* (New York: Broadway Books, 2007).

232. Allen Luks, *The Healing Power of Doing Good: The Health and Spiritual Benefits of Helping Others* (New York: Fawcett Columbine, 1991).

233. Sharon Salzburg, *Lovingkindness: the Revolutionary Art of Happiness* (Boston: Shambala, 1995).

234. Bernie Siegel, *Peace, Love and Healing: Bodymind Communication & The Path To Self-Healing: An Exploration* (New York: Harper & Row, 1990) 30-32.

235. Shel Silverstein, *The Missing Piece* (New York: HarperCollins, 1976).

236. L Giles et al., "Effect of social networks on 10 year survival in very old Australians: the Australian longitudinal study of aging," *Journal of Epidemiology and Community Health*, 59 (2005): 574-79.

237. M McPherson et al., "Social Isolation in America: Changes in Core Discussion Networks over Two Decades," *American Sociological Review*, 71 (2006): 353-75.

238. S Pressman, S Cohen, et al., "Loneliness, Social Network Size, and Immune Response to Influenza Vaccination in College Freshman," *Health Psychology*, 24 (2005): 297-306.

239. Y Michael et al., "Health behaviors, social networks, and healthy aging: Cross-sectional evidence from the Nurses' health Study," *Quality of Life Research*, 8 (1999): 711-22.

240. In *Men's Health*, April (2008). For further reading see the book: Michael McCullough, *Beyond Revenge: The Evolution of the Forgiveness Instinct* (San Francisco: Josey-Bass, 2008).

241. Kathleen Brehony, *Living a Connected Life: Creating and maintaining Relationships That Last* (New York: Henry Holt and Company, 2003).

242. L Giles et al., "Effect of social networks on 10 year survival in very old Australians: the Australian longitudinal study of aging," *Journal of Epidemiology and Community Health*, 59 (2005): 574-79.

243. J Turner-Cobb et al., "Social Support and Salivary Cortisol in Women With Metastatic Breast Cancer," *Psychosomatic Medicine*, 62 (2000): 337-45.

244. Henry Dreher, *The Immune Power Personality: 7 Traits You Can Develop to Stay Healthy* (New York: Plume, 1996).

245. D Shrock et al., "Effects of a Psychosocial Intervention on Survival Among Patients with Stage I Breast and Prostate Cancer: A Matched Case-Control Study," *Alternative Therapies in Health and Medicine*, 5 (1999): 49-55.

246. Online groups such as PatientsLikeMe share information and offer support for folks seeking out networking opportunities without leaving the house. www.patientslikeme.com/.

247. Multiple sources: M Speca et al., "A Randomized, Wait-List Controlled Clinical Trial: The Effect of Mindfulness Meditation-Based Stress Reduction Program on Mood and Symptoms of Stress in Cancer Outpatients," *Psychosomatic Medicine*, 62 (2000): 613-22. R Baer, "Mindfulness Training as a clinical intervention: A conceptual and empirical review," *Clinical Psychology: Science and Practice*, 10 (2006): 125-43. N Allen et al., "Mindfulness-based psychotherapies: a review of conceptual foundations, empirical evidence and practical considerations," *Australian and New Zealand Journal of Psychiatry*, 40 (2006): 285-94. R Davidson et al., "Alterations in Brain and Immune Function Produced by Mindfulness Meditation," *Psychosomatic Medicine*, 65 (2003): 564-70. P Grossman et al., "Mindfulness-based stress reductions and health benefits: A meta-analysis," *Journal of Psychosomatic Research*, 57 (2004): 35-43.

248. M Bambling, "Mind, Body, and Heart: Psychotherapy and the Relationship between Mental and Physical Health," *Psychotherapy in Australia*, 12 (2006): 52-59.

249. Jon Kabat-Zinn, *Full Catastrophe Living: Using the Wisdom of Your Body and Mind to Face Stress, Pain and Illness* (New York: Dell Publishing, 1990).

250. E Rossi, "Stress-induced alternative gene splicing in mind-body medicine," *Advances in Mind-Body Medicine*, 20 (2004): 12-9

251. R Davidson et al., "Alterations in Brain and Immune Function Produced by Mindfulness Meditation," *Psychosomatic Medicine*, 65 (2003): 564-70.

Chapter Nine

252. Wikipedia, "Ignaz Semmelweis," en.wikipedia.org/wiki/Semmelweis.

253. S Wolf, "Effects of Suggestion and Conditioning on the Action of Chemical Agents in Human Subjects; The Pharmacology of Placebos", *Journal of Clinical Investigation*, 29 (1950): 100–109.

254. J Moskowitz et al., "Positive Affect uniquely Predicts Lower Risk of Mortality in People with Diabetes," *Health Psychology*, 27 (2008): S73-S82.

255. Ibid.

256. Ibid.

257. A Edmundson, "Aging Well May Mean 'Mind Over Matter.'" *WebMD Health News*, Dec 16 (2005): www.webmd.com/healthy-aging/news/20051216/aging-well-may-mean-mind-over-matter.

258. L Kubzansky et al., "Is the Glass Half Empty or Half Full? A Prospective Study of Optimism and Coronary Heart Disease in the Normative Aging Study." *Psychosomatic Medicine*, 63 (2001): 910-916.

259. M Mondloch et al., "Does how you do depend on how you think you'll do? A systematic review of the evidence for a relation between patients' recovery expectations and health outcomes," *Canadian Medical Association Journal*, 165 (2001): 174-9.

260. Multiple sources: E Giltay, "Dispositional Optimism and the Risk of Cardiovascular Death: The Zutphen Elderly Study," *Archives of Internal Medicine*, 166 (2006): 413-36. Also E Giltay et al., Optimism and All-Cause and Cardiovascular Mortality in a Prospective Cohort of Elderly Dutch Men and Women," *Archives of General Psychiatry*, 61 (2004): 1126-35. Also M Lemonick and A Park/Mankato, "The Nun Study," *Time*, May 14 (2001): www.time.com/time/magazine/article/0,9171,999867,00.html.

261. T Maruta et al. "Optimism-pessimism assessed in the 1960s and self-reported health status 30 years later," *Mayo Clinic Proceedings*, 77 (2002): 748-753.

262. D Danner, D Snowden et al., "Positive Emotions in Early Life & Longevity: Findings from the Nun Study," *Journal of Personality and Social Psychology*, 80 (2001): 804-813. Also D Snowdon et al., "Linguistic ability in early life and cognitive function and Alzheimer's disease in late life. Findings from the Nun Study," *JAMA*, 275 (1996): 528-32.

263. J Pennebaker and L Stone, "Words of Wisdom: Language Use Over the Life Span," *Journal of Personality and Social Psychology*. 85 (2003): 291-301.

264. Martin Seligman, *Authentic Happiness: Using the New Positive Psychology to Realize Your Potential for Lasting Fulfillment* (New York: The Free Press, 2002).

265. Emmett Miller, *Deep Healing: The Essence of Mind/Body Medicine* (Carlsbad, CA: Hay House, 1997): 70.

266. E Schoenhofen et al., "Characteristics of 32 Supercentenarians," *Journal of the American Geriatrics Society*, 54 (2006): 1237-40.

267. E Giltay et al., "Dispositional Optimism and All-Cause and Cardiovascular Mortality in a Prospective Cohort of Elderly Dutch Men and Women," *Archives of General Psychiatry*, 61 (2004): 1126-35.

268. Harold Kushner, *When Bad Things Happen to Good People* (New York: Avon Books, 1981).

269. J Pennebaker and C Chung, "Expressive Writing, Emotional Upheavals, and Health" in *Handbook of Health Psychology*, ed. Howard Friedman and Roxane Silver (New York: Oxford University Press, 2007): 263-84.

270. M Quinlan, "Using Our Midlife Mojo," *More Magazine*, Dec/Jan (2005/2006): 59-60.

271. J Lackner et al., "Self-Administered Cognitive Behavior Therapy for Moderate to Severe Irritable Bowel Syndrome: Clinical Efficacy, Tolerability, Feasability," *Clinical Gastroenterology and Hepatology*, 6 (2008): 899-906.

272. S Levy, R Herberman, J Rodin and M Seligman, "Psychological and immunological effects of a randomized psychosocial treatment trial for colon cancer and malignant melanoma patients," in *Conceptual and Methodological Issues in Cancer Psychotherapy Intervention Studies*, ed. H Balner and Y van Rood (Amsterdam: Swets & Zeitlinger Publishers, 1990).

273. Helen Mrosla, "All the Good Things," in *Chicken Soup for the Soul*, ed. Jack Canfield and Mark Victor Hansen (Deerfield Beach, Fl: Health Communications, Inc., 2001).

Chapter Ten

274. Claudia Wallace, "Unlocking Pain's Secrets," *Time*, June 11 (1984).

275. Victor Frankl, *Man's Search for Meaning* (Boston: Beacon, 2006): 112.

276. Kathleen Brehony, *After the Darkest Hour: How Suffering Begins the Journey to Wisdom* (New York: Henry Holt and Company, 2000).

277. Robert Ader et al., *Psychoneuroimmunology* (New York: Academic Press, 1991): 1120.

ACKNOWLEDGMENTS

My profound appreciation to Dr. Gerald Goldklang of Georgia Cancer Treatment and Hematology Center, whose great belief in this work inspired him to generously provide this six-week program for his patients and others in the community for more than a decade. The honor has been mine. Each group brings an abundance of good things into my life, and it is my privilege to learn from each and every one. My heartfelt gratitude is beyond measure for the love and patience the long-term group has shown me over the years—we've been through a lot together, and I thank you.

Shaping this program is the cumulative wisdom of my many teachers, without whom this book would not have been possible. Too numerous to mention in total, I will list only a few influential in my own recovery: Albert Marchetti, M.D., whose clear and relevant work led me to Rita Stucky, Ph.D., of the Menninger Clinic, who taught me with amazing grace and skill not only how to breathe but to rethink the nature of health and illness. After reading the eye-opening books by Bernie Siegel, M.D., I called the organization he founded, ECaP, and was referred to Getting Well, a behavioral medicine program in Orlando, Florida. It was founded by Deirdre Brigham and Philip Toal, whose work over the years impacted the lives of countless participants. Deirdre became my friend, mentor, and closest ally on my healing journey. I owe her more than I could ever express and miss her unfathomably. As their clinical assistant, I met patients who added their own unique stamp to this work and to whom I remain indebted. Our board of directors at Getting Well read like a Who's Who of psychoneuroimmunology, including Lawrence LeShan, whose books helped chart my course (for fresh inspiration I periodically reread his classic work, *Cancer as a Turning Point*).

Many others have brought me priceless gifts of wisdom, inspiration, and encouragement and are named in the text and reflected in the Resource Guide.

Later, by stroke of timing and location, I became the program director at ECaP, where I am most grateful to Dr. Andrew Salner, chief oncologist at the Helen and Harry Gray Cancer Center, a gracious and dedicated physician who first believed in the program enough to provide it without charge to patients.

Without all the research, though, this program would just be another good idea. This work stands on the shoulders of the many health professionals, researchers, and scientists recognized throughout the pages of this book who so willingly shared their work, ideas, and experiences and took the time to respond to my queries. The evidence they provide underscores each and every concept or idea herein, and I am indebted to their accumulated knowledge, the questions they pose, and the way they go about seeking the answers.

Special thanks to faculty advisors Drs. Anne Webster, Peggy Wright, and Liz Blumberg for their lovely words and encouragement after reading an early draft. Literature professor and writer Michael Datcher and his wife, author Jenoyne Adams, were incredibly supportive, but if it weren't for my mother warning that the book was going to be published posthumously, it might never have happened. Kathleen Brehony was essential to the process. She was there in the beginning, coaching and cheering me on, and later when the real work heated up, she was my champion and guide. Her remarkable expertise is reflected throughout. All of which led me to Jill Marsal of the Sandra Dijkstra Agency, whose belief in the project from the first moment she saw it carried us through, even as the fires in San Bernardino forced her to evacuate her home. I am particularly grateful to Connie Shaw and Scott Perrizo of Sentient Publications, whose passion and belief made this book possible and who are a pleasure to work with.

Key to meeting my publishing deadline was the honor of a Hambidge Fellowship, which I was delighted to receive. The luxury of ample solitude for reflection and research was priceless. My many thanks to the residency program, its board of directors, the executive director, Judy Morris Lampert, and the residency director, Bob Thomas, for providing the support and setting for creative work (and for all the culinary pleasures that graced my evenings).

Numerous friends and family offered amazing support and performed many acts of loving-kindness in behalf of this project. To name them all might seem like a bad night at the Oscar's so I'm confining myself to those who worked directly on the manuscript itself: June Stockdale, who eliminated commas from the page faster than I could type them; Patricia Pirkle Coury and Nancie Talley, excellent writers in their own right, who went far beyond the call of friendship in providing a steady stream of support, encouragement and editorial advice (along with saltines, flashlights, puzzles, coasters, and whistles).

Most of all, I thank my partner and best friend, tireless reader and champion supporter: my husband, Michael Milton. His medical insight and expertise, keen eye and superb wit sharpened and refined every page. Without his absolute encouragement and insistence that this book happen, I'd still be writing chapter 2. And last but certainly not least, a hearty acknowledgement to my beautiful, loving, funny, and neurotic co-author, The Great Dog Sandy, who often sat in my lap while I typed and thinks everything I do is just the best.

PERMISSIONS

Page 119: From The Healing Power of Sound, by Mitchell L. Gaynor, M.D., © 1999 by Mitchell L. Gaynor, M.D. Reprinted by arrangement with Shambhala Publications Inc., Boston, MA. www.shambhala.com.

Page 148: "Things to Think" from *Morning Poems* by Robert Bly. Copyright © 1997 by Robert Bly. Reprinted by permission of HarperCollins Publishers.

Page 168: Helen Keller quotation from *The Story of My Life* courtesy of the American Foundation for the Blind, Helen Keller Archives. Used with permission.

Page 189-90: Pearsall, Paul. *Super Immunity.* © 1987 The McGraw Hill Companies. Reprinted with permission of The McGraw Hill Companies.

Page 201-2: The Resiliency Quiz is reprinted with permission from *The Resiliency Advantage* by Al Siebert, PhD. © Copyright 2005, Al Siebert, PhD.

Pages 210-11: Pages 30-32 from Peace, Love and Healing by Bernie S. Siegel, M.D. Copyright © 1989 by Bernard S. Siegel, M.D. Preprinted by permission of HarperCollins Publishers.

Pages 249-50: Helen P. Mrosla, excerpt from "All the Good Things" from *Chicken Soup for the Soul,* edited by Jack Canfield and Mark Victor Hansen. Originally published in *Proteus: A Journal of Ideas* (Spring 1991). Reprinted with the permission of Health Communications, Inc., www. hcibooks.com.

INDEX

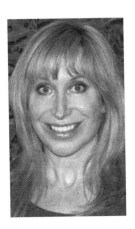

ABOUT THE AUTHOR

Brenda Stockdale is the Director of Behavioral Medicine at Radiotherapy Clinics of Georgia (a Vantage Oncology affiliate), and a nationally recognized pioneer in the practical application of psychoneuroimmunology. Her programs are endorsed by leading specialists and have been implemented in hospitals, cancer centers and primary care practices. She has also been the National Program Director for the cancer support organization founded by best-selling author and surgeon Bernie Siegel, MD.

Stockdale has been featured on *The Oprah Winfrey Show*, NPR, ABC radio and in a variety of print media, including *Bottom Line Health, Good Housekeeping, 'O' The Oprah Magazine* and *Natural Health*.

Her 6-week program, outlined in her recent book, *You Can Beat the Odds*, has been praised by Harvard scientists, physicians and epidemiologists "as a prescription, in and of itself, for maximizing one's health" and "*the* health book to read this year."

She developed a groundbreaking health psychology program for primary care settings specializing in preventive medicine, autoimmunity, and stress-related conditions. A leader in her field, she has taught, presented workshops, lectured nationally over the last fifteen years for a variety of corporate and special interest groups, authored scholarly articles and book chapters for academic texts, and co-authored an integrative medicine newsletter. She is a clinician in the field of behavioral medicine, but it is her own experience with life-altering and catastrophic illness that anchors the subject in an intimate way.

Sentient Publications, LLC publishes books on cultural creativity, experimental education, transformative spirituality, holistic health, new science, ecology, and other topics, approached from an integral viewpoint. Our authors are intensely interested in exploring the nature of life from fresh perspectives, addressing life's great questions, and fostering the full expression of the human potential. Sentient Publications' books arise from the spirit of inquiry and the richness of the inherent dialogue between writer and reader.

Our Culture Tools series is designed to give social catalyzers and cultural entrepreneurs the essential information, technology, and inspiration to forge a sustainable, creative, and compassionate world.

We are very interested in hearing from our readers. To direct suggestions or comments to us, or to be added to our mailing list, please contact:

SENTIENT PUBLICATIONS, LLC
1113 Spruce Street
Boulder, CO 80302
303-443-2188
contact@sentientpublications.com
www.sentientpublications.com

24741577R00191

Made in the USA
Middletown, DE
04 October 2015